Current Topics in Pathology

Ergebnisse der Pathologie

Edited by

E. Grundmann · **W. H. Kirsten**
Münster *Chicago*

Advisory Board

Volume 57

With 80 Figures

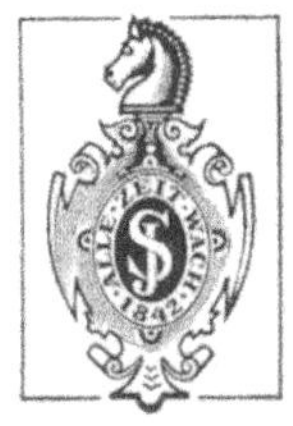

Springer-Verlag Berlin · Heidelberg · New York 1973

ISBN-13: 978-3-642-65467-1   e-ISBN-13: 978-3-642-65465-7
DOI: 10.1007/978-3-642-65465-7

Contents

List of Contributors

Solange G. abuNassar, Beekman Downtown Hospital, 170 William Street, New York, NY 10037, USA

Henry A. Azar, Veterans Administration Hospital, 13000 North 30th Street, Tampa, FL 33612, USA

J. Steven McDougal, Columbia-Presbyterian Medical Center, 622-630 West 168th Street, New York, NY 10032, USA

M. Mendelovici, Universidad de Los Andes, Apartado 75, Mérida, Venezuela

J. Moppert, I. Medizinische Klinik der Universität, Bürgerspital, CH-4000 Basel, Switzerland

Edward A. Moscovic, Harlem Hospital Center, 136th Street and Lenox Avenue, New York, NY 10038, USA

Herwart F. Otto, Pathologisches Institut der Universität, D-2000 Hamburg-20, Martinistraße 52, Germany

Hanspeter Rohr, Pathologisches Institut der Universität, Schönbeinstraße 40, CH-4056 Basel, Switzerland

K. Salfelder, Instituto de Anatomia Patologica, Universidad de Los Andes, Apartado 75, Mérida, Venezuela

J. Schwarz, Clinical Laboratories, Jewish Hospital, Cincinnati, OH 45229, USA

G. Thiel, Medizinische Universitätsklinik, Bürgerspital, CH-4000 Basel, Switzerland

Hans Ulrich Zollinger, Pathologisches Institut der Universität, Schönbeinstraße 40, CH-4056 Basel Switzerland

From the Department of Pathology and Medicine: University of Basle, Switzerland

Morphology and Pathogenesis of Glomerulopathy in Cadaver Kidney Allografts Treated with Antilymphocyte Globulin*

(Clinical, Light, Electron and Immunofluorescent Optic Examinations)

H. U. ZOLLINGER, J. MOPPERT, G. THIEL, H.-P. ROHR

With 42 Figures

Contents

Severe glomerular changes occuring in long-surviving kidney transplants have been known for some years. Several authors have interpreted them as glomerulonephritis (lit. cf. HUME *et al.*, 1970, MILGROM *et al.*, 1971). The present paper intends to mainly clarify the light-, electron- and immunofluorescent-optic morphology, and to decide whether it could be glomerulonephritis. Besides, we were interested in the correlation between transplant glomerulopathy (TGP) and clinical findings. Finally, we tried to clarify the pathogenesis of this peculiar TGP and looked for some causal relationship to antilymphocytic globulin (ALG) treatment.

A. Material and Method

21 cases of patients with cadaver kidney transplants were evaluated by 30 kidney punctates and 7 kidney slices. Cases 3 and 19 were examined immediately post mortem; in patients 2, 9, 17, 18 and 21 nephrectomy specimens were at hand. All cases were examined in paraffin (HE, PAS, Picro-Mallory, CAB, Giemsa, methenamine-silver staining) and semithin sections (azur eosin)

---

* Supported by Swiss National Foundation for Scientific Research No. 3—307.70

by light and electron microscopy: Kidney tissue was split into small tissue blocks, fixed in phosphate-buffered glutardialdehyde (3 %, pH 7,25) and post-fixed in osmium tetroxide (2 %); then embedded in Epon (Epikote 812). Reichert Ultratom OmU2 was used for sectioning. Ultrathin sections were stained with uranyl acetate and lead citrate. A Zeiss electronmicroscope type 9A was available for electron microscopic examination.

The essential changes, etc. are shown in Table 1, whereas the relations between degree of severity, space of time after transplantation and ALG treatment are depicted in Fig. 1.

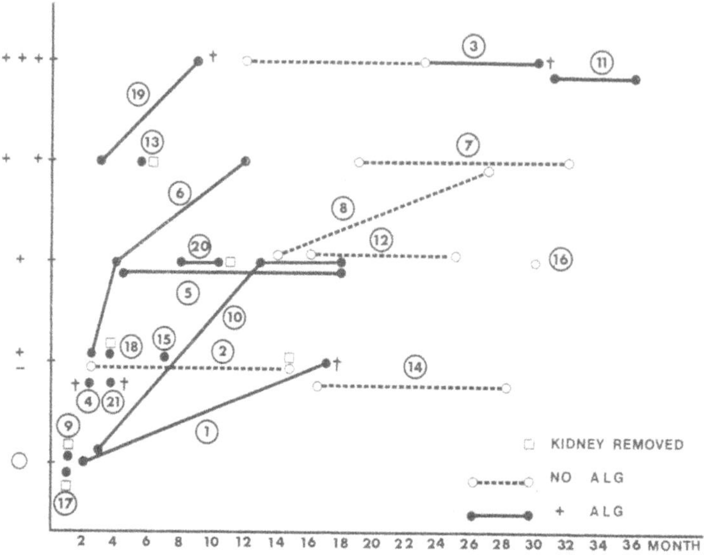

Fig. 1. Relations between grade of severity of transplant glomerulopathy (0 — + + +), space of time after transplantation and antilymphocytic globulin (ALG) treatment. Compare case numbers with tables 1 and 2

We examined 32 biopsies of 20 patients by immunofluorescence-histology (s. Table 2). No material was available in case 13 and the first biopsy of cases 1, 2, 3, and 12. Processing: Incubation for 30 min in a moist at room temperature of airdried kryostat sections with rabbit-immune sera (Behring, Germany): 7S specific antihuman IgG–IgM, also antihuman β1C (C'3), anti-human fibrin and anti-horse-gammaglobulin. After thorough washing of the preparations, second incubation with FITC marked pig-anti-rabbit-gamma-globulin (Sevac, Prague). After repeated washings, evaluation by Wild M 20 microscope by means of blue-light fluorescence. As controls served sections of a normal human kidney which, due to technical reasons, could not be transplanted.

In 12 out of 22 examined cadaver kidney transplants (21 recipients) histo-compatibility was tested by means of lymphocyte typing. A modification of Terasaki's method of microcyte toxicity was applied (Jeannet et al., 1969/70).

Table 1. Presentation of cases (for immunhistology see Table 2)

Column 3: Fabry = morbus Fabry, Gl.n. = glomerulonephritis, Py.n. = pyelonephritis, i.n. = non destructive interstitial nephritis, m.G.l.n. = membranous glomerulonephritis, m.n.s. = malignant nephrosclerosis.

Column 4: a = histocompatibility ranks of RAPAPORT and DAUSSET (1969).
b = clinical histocompatibility classification (see text).

Column 5: file number of punction.

Column 6: time since transplantation: d = days, w = weeks, m = months.

Column 7: Creatinine clearance (ml/min.).

Column 8: Antilymphocytic serum therapy: 1 = stop 10 months after transpl, 2 = since 4 months only intramuscularly, 3 = since 10 months only muscularly, 4 = total 40 ml for three days after transpl., 5 = stop $3^1/_2$ months after transpl., 6 = stop 5 months after transpl., 7 = stop $4^1/_2$ months after transpl.

Column 9: X-ray treatment.

Column 11: Degree of severity of TGP: $\emptyset$ = no conspicuous change; $\pm$ = slight changes; $+$ = distinct TGP; $++$ = rather severe degree of TGP; $+++$ = extremely severe degree.

Column 12: Osmiophilic deposits: c = incapsular BM, s = subendothelial, m = mesangial.

Column 13: d, w, m see column 6; nephrectomy because of: v.r. = vascular rejection, s.r. = spontaneous rupture of transpl. kidney, a.h. = arterial haemorrhage, n.u. = necrosis of ureter, a.r. = acute rejection.

1	2	3	4		5	6	7	8	9	10	11	12	13
Case	Age Sex	Prim. disease	Histocomp. a Rank	b Clin.	Pct.	Time since transpl.	Ccr.	ALG	Rö.	Prot. uria mg/die	Glomerulo- pathia	Osmioph. depots	Katamnesis
1	38, ♂	Fabry	—	B	276	$6^1/_2$ m	42	$\emptyset$	900 R	45	$\emptyset$	c $+$	s. Pect. 400
	38, ♂	Fabry	—	B	400	$16^1/_2$ m	8,3	$+$	900 R	289	$\pm$	s $++$	† $16^1/_2$ m: nocardia pneumonia
2	35, ♀	Gl.n.	—	C	330	6 w	25	$\emptyset$	1200 R	720	$\pm$	$\emptyset$	s. Pct. 420
	35, ♀	Gl.n.	—	C	420	14 m	0	$+^1$	1200 R	8800	$\pm$	s $+$	v. r. 14 m
3	46, ♀	Gl.n.	—	B	342	12 m	44	$\emptyset$	$\emptyset$	598	$+++$	$\emptyset$	s. Pct. 490
	46, ♀	Gl.n.	—	B	416	23 m	39	$\emptyset$	$\emptyset$	4450	$+++$	$\emptyset$	s. Pct. 490
	46, ♀	Gl.n.	—	B	490	30 m	9	$+$	$\emptyset$	2000	$+++$	$\emptyset$	† 30 m: liver dystrophy

1	2	3	4		5	6	7	8	9	10	11	12	13
Case	Age Sex	Prim. disease	Histocomp. a Rank	b Clin.	Pct.	Time since transpl.	Ccr.	ALG	Rö.	Prot. uria mg/die	Glomerulo-pathia	Osmioph. depots	Katamnesis
4	29, ♀	Py.n.	8	C	409	50 d	7,4	+	450 R	1120	±	∅	a.r.: 51 D; † 9 m: influenza p neumonia
5	24, ♂	i.n.	9	B	422	10 w	40	+	450 R	280	+	∅	functioning
	24, ♂	i.n.	9	B	614	19 m	34	+	450 R	280	+	m+	functioning
6	46, ♀	i.n.	5	B	468	30 d	8,8	+	450 R	650	±	c+	functioning
	46, ♀	i.n.	5	B	520	6 m	37	+[2]	450 R	150	+	c+	functioning
	46, ♀	i.n.	5	B	597	11½ m	26	+[3]	450 R	560	±	∅	functioning
7	27, ♂	Gl.n.	—	A$_2$	459	19 m	73	∅	450 R	315	++	s++ m+ c+	functioning
	27, ♂	Gl.n.	—	A$_2$	619	32 m	62	∅	450 R	825	++	m++ s++	functioning
8	40, ♂	Gl.n.	—	A$_2$	498	14½ m	75	+[4]	600 R	3100	+	∅	functioning
	40, ♂	Gl.n.	—	A$_2$	660	27 m	72	+[4]	600 R	2500	++	∅	functioning
9	47, ♂	Gl.n.	6	C	519	7 d	0	+	∅	?	∅	m++	v.r. 1 o d, sec. transpl.
10	47, ♂	Py.n.	8	B	411	7 w	86	+	750 R	580	∅	∅	functioning
	47, ♂	Py.n.	8	B	522	13 m	50	+	750 R	2900	+	s++	functioning
	47, ♂	Py.n.	8	B	594	18 m	43	+	750 R	4700	+	∅	functioning
11	36, ♀	Gl.n. +diab.	—	B	523	31 m	16	+	∅	780	+++	s+	functioning
	36, ♀	Gl.n. +diab.	—	B	591	36 m	5,4	+	∅	900 −10500	+++	s++	v.r. 49 m, † 49 m thrombocytopenia

12	44, ♀ Gl.n.	—	A_1	546	16 m	73	∅	450 R	216	+	∅	functioning
	44, ♀ Gl.n.	—	A_1	571	25 m	95	∅	450 R	460	+	∅	functioning
13	45, ♂ m.Gl.n.	—	C	410	5½ m	42	+	300 R	625	++	m++	v.r. 6½ M
14	45, ♂ Gl.n.	—	A_1	547	16½ m	63	∅	450 R	140	±	m+	functioning
	45, ♂ Gl.n.	—	A_1	604	28 m	64	∅	450 R	75	±	m±	functioning
15	34, ♂ i.N.	2	A_1	566	8 m	97	+[5]	∅	1080	±	m++	functioning
16	40, ♂ Gl.n.		A_1	581	30 m	85	∅	600 R	2000	±	∅	functioning
17	46, ♂ Py.n.	4	∅	595	8 d	0	+	450 R	?	∅	∅	s.r. 8 d
18	47, ♂ Gl.n.?	3	0	582	34 d	70	+	∅	325	±	∅	a.h. 34 d
19	24, ♀ Gl.n.	6	C	605	3½ m	40	+	1050 R	850	++	∅	s.Pct. 677
	24, ♀ Gl.n.	6	C	677	9 m	0	+[6]	1050 R	?	+++	0	v.r. 9 m † pyocyaneus septicemia
20	47, ♀ Py.n.	4	B	611	7 m	57	+[7]	750 R	144	+	∅	functioning
	47, ♀ Py.n.	4	B	634	9 m	54	+[7]	750 R	140	+	∅	v.r. 9 m
21	50, ♂ m.n.s.	5	C	635	10 w	0	+	350 R	130	±	∅	n.u. 3 m † 4½ m cardial insufficiency

Table 2. Immunofluorescent findings

IG: Immunoglobulins. C′3:β1C/1A. Fi: Fibrin(ogen). ALG: Horse antilymphocyte globulin. OSI: Overall severity of immunofluorescent findings *irrespective* of ALG-depositions. Intraglomerular localization: me: mesangial, p: along the periphery of glomerular capillary loops (i.e. basement membrane), mep: combination of me and p., cl: within glomerular capillary lumina.

Pattern of glomerular fluorescence: f: focal, d: diffuse. Amount of fluorescence:

∅   = negative.
+   = less than 30 % of structures positive; slight.
++   = 30—60 % of structures positive; moderate.
+++   = over 60 % of structures positive; marked.
*) = immunofluorescent pattern of nephrotoxic plus complex-type nephritis induced by ALG.

Table 2a:

Case N.	Biopsy N.	IG	C′3	Fi	ALG	OSI
1	276	Immunofluorescent microscopy not done				
1	400	mep f +	p f ++ p d +	mep f +	p f ++ p d +	+
2	330	Immunofluorescent microscopy not done				
2	420	∅	∅	∅	p f ++	∅
3	342	Immunofluorescent microscopy not done				
3	416	mep f ++	mep f ++	mep f +++	∅	+++
3	490	mep f ++	mep f +	mep f +	mep f ++	+++
4	409	mep f +	∅	mep f +	p d +++	+
5	422	me f +	p d ++	∅	p d +++	+
5	614	me f +	me f +	∅	p d +++	+
6	468	∅	p d +++	∅	p d +++	∅
6	520	∅	∅	∅	p d +++	∅
6	597	∅	∅	∅	p d +++	∅
7	459	mep f ++	mep f ++	∅	∅	++
7	619	mep f ++	mep f ++	me f +	∅	+++
8	498	me f ++	me f +	∅	∅	+
8	660	me f +	me f +	∅	∅	+
9	519	∅	∅	cl f +	p d +++	∅

Initially, 13 HL-A-antigens were tested. Subsequently the number was gradually increased to 24 (Jeannet et al., 1971). According to Rapaport and Dausset (1970) HL-A-compatibility was assessed in ranks 1–15.

The role of HL-A histocompatibility between non-related donors is controversial. Therefore, in addition, the degree of histocompatibility was retro-

Table 2b:

Case N.	Pct. nr.	IG	Immunofluorescent findings II			
			C'3	Fi	ALG	OSI
10	411	me f ++	∅	me f +	p d +++	+
10	522	∅	∅	∅	p d +++	∅
10	594	p d +++ p f ++	∅	∅	p d +++ p f ++*)	
11	523	mep f ++	mep f ++	mep f +	mep f ++	+++
11	591	mep f ++	mep f ++	cl f +	mep f ++	+++
12	546	Immunofluorescent microscopy not done				
12	571	mep f +	mep f +	∅	∅	+
13	410	Immunofluorescent microscopy not done				
14	547	mep f +	mep f +	mep f +	∅	+
14	604	mep f ++	mep f ++	me f +	∅	+
15	566	∅	∅	∅	p d +++	∅
16	581	mep f ++	mep f +	mep f +	∅	++
17	595	∅	∅	∅	p d +++	∅
18	582	∅	∅	∅	p d +++	∅
19	605	me f ++	me f ++	∅	p d +++ me f ++	++
19	677	mep f ++	mep f ++	∅	mep f ++	++
20	611	me f +	me f +	∅	p d +++	+
20	634	me f +	∅	∅	p d +++	+
21	635	∅	∅	∅	p d +++	∅

spectively rated by the clinical course. 4 ranks of clinical compatibility were distinguished:

O = non-assessable because of a too short course or non-immunologic reasons of failure.

A = good clinical compatibility, i.e. course without any signs of rejection (A_1), or only 1–2 acute rejection episodes easily influenced by therapy without further tendency of relapse (A_2).

B = 1 or more severe rejection episodes which could be brought under control only with difficulties.

C = irreversible acute, subacute or quickly progressing chronic rejection, unaffectable by therapy.

All patients were treated with the standard dosage of azothioprine and prednisone. 14 cases additionally received antilymphocytic globulin (ALG) i.v. (Thiel, 1969). In patient 11 azothioprine was stopped 7 months before the first, and 12 months before the second biopsy. During this time, she received only ALG i.v. and a small dosage of prednisone (0–15 mg daily).

The kidney biopsies were chiefly carried out percutaneously with a modified Silverman needle. Proteinuria was measured in the 24-h-urine by Kjeldahl's method of protein analysis; its values were given in mg protein per 24 hs. Table 1 lists the proteinuria of each patient at the time of the kidney biopsy.

B. Findings
1. Light and Electron Microscopy

In light microscopy (Fig. 2) only moderately severe and severe degrees of TGP show an enlarged mesangium and a thickened basement membrane (BM). In semithin sections, the picture of the severe changes reminds of membranous glomerulonephritis (Fig. 3). Silver staining, however, often shows a duplication of the BM; spikes on the external membrane are lacking (Fig. 4). In cases of extremely severe lesions, the loops are often heavily narrowed by the thickened BM. An increase in the number of cells can be demonstrated neither in the mesangium, nor in the endothelium, nor in the capsular epithelium (exception: case 3, s. below).

Glomerular changes, caused by collapse, can regularly be found in cases with severe vascular involvement (cases 1, 2, 4, 9). The BM of the loops is profusely undulated; the loops have collapsed (Fig. 5). Furthermore, these cases show scattered, completely hyalinized glomerula. Mixtures of collapse and TGP were often observed.

Electron microscopy shows the *glomerular basement membrane* thickened in all cases of TGP (Fig. 6). Stronger magnification reveals that the external lamina rara, as well as the lamina densa, ordinarily do not indicate deviation from normal. Only in cases of vascularly triggered collapse of the loops the entire BM is thickened, whereby mainly the lamina densa seems to be enlarged (Fig. 7). — In a very severe grade of TGP it is often difficult to determine the exact boundary between lamina densa and internal lamina rara. The impression, that the lamina densa is distinctly narrowed under these circumstances, is evident (Fig. 8).

The main changes of TGP occur in the internal lamina rara. We observed the first changes in this series of cases after $1^1/_2$ months (cases 2, 4, 6) (Fig. 1). They consist in finely granular electron-lucent thickenings of the internal lamina rara. In relation to a given loop, the change may be rather diffuse, or nodular (Figs. s. 9–11). Apart from loosely arranged finest osmiophilic granula (Fig. 10, 12, 13, 19, 20), an actual structure of this loosened internal lamina rara can, even at high magnification, not be recognized. In 5 cases, we found osmiophilic filaments in it; this may be fibrin, split or in the process of splitting (Fig. 21).

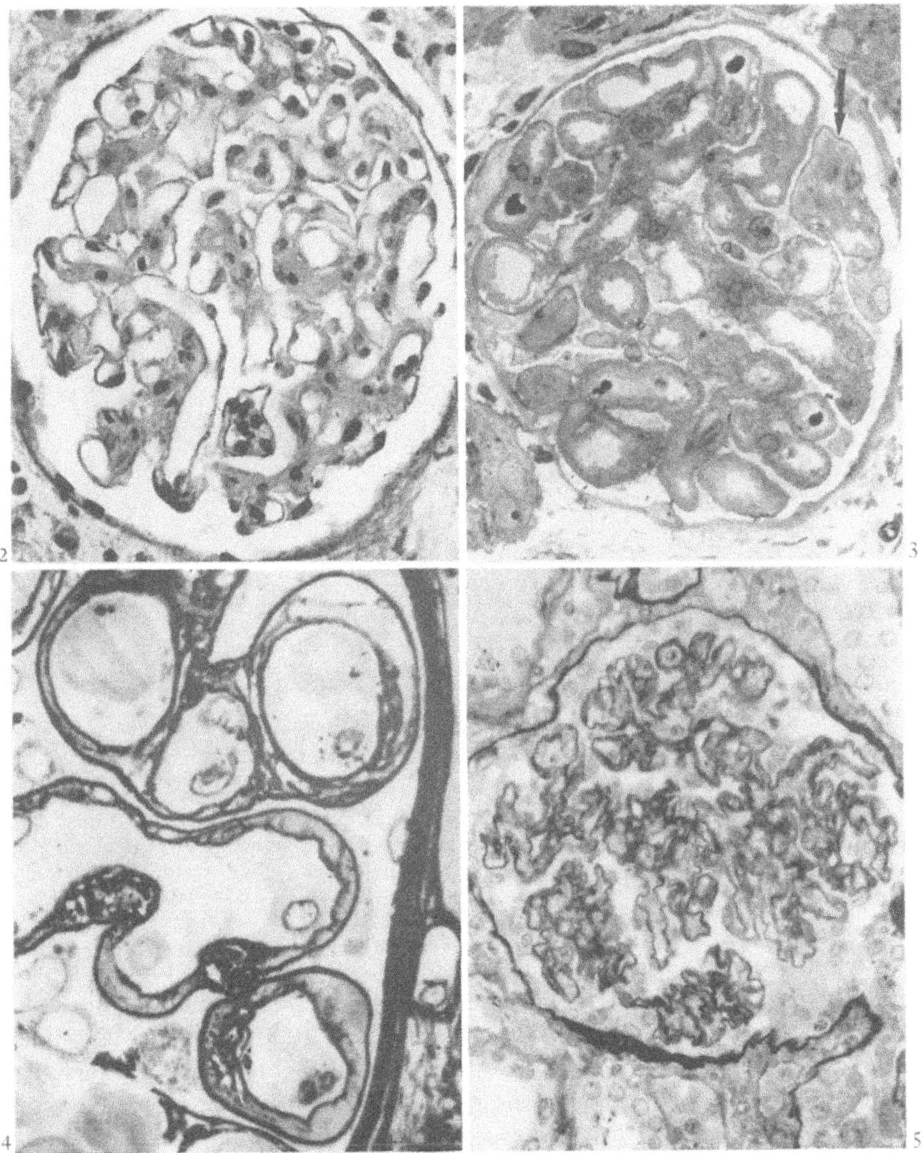

Fig. 2. TGP grade $++$, $3^1/_2$ months after transplantation (case 19). Thickening of the walls of some glomerular loops, increase of mesangial area without nuclear proliferation. PAS, 375 ×

Fig. 3. Very distinct TGP, $2^1/_2$ years after transplantation (case 11). Greatly thickened capillary walls, no proliferation of cells. One capillary lumen almost blocked (→). Semithin section, azur eosin staining, 375 ×

Fig. 4. Same case as Fig. 3, $^1/_2$ year later (3 years after transpl.). Distinct duplication of the basement membrane, optically empty space between the two layers. Semithin section, methenamine-silver staining, 1 200 ×

Fig. 5. Collaps of glomerular loops, undulation of BM, $5^1/_2$ months after transplantation (case 13). PAS, 440 ×

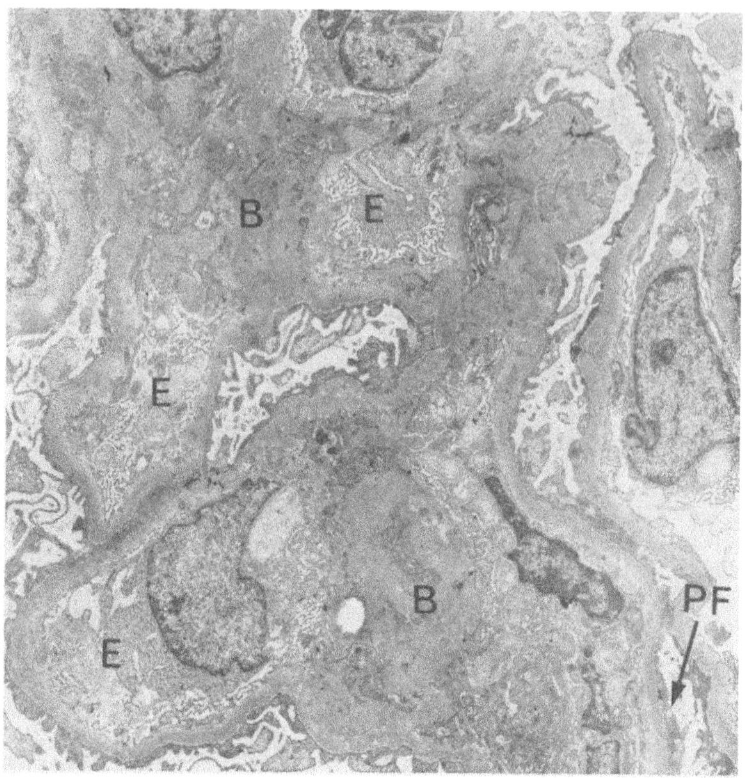

Fig. 6. Electronmicroscopic photograph of a typical TGP, 9 months after transplantation (case 20). Thickened BM. Garland-shaped arcades of endothelium (E) are almost completely the lumina of the loops. Basement membrane-like substance (B) of the mesangium much increased without multiplication of the nuclei, focal pedicle fusion (PF). 3 570 ×

More frequently, cell constituents, consisting partly of cytoplasmic constituents, only enclosed by a membrane (Fig. 14), can be found in this thickened internal lamina rara; partly, however, genuine endothelial invaginations, extending into this loosened area, can be recognized (Fig. 15). At a very high degree of TGP these cell inclusions may become huge. Scattered mesangial cells seem to creep under the lamina densa into the region of the thickened lamina rara (Fig. 8). At subsequent phases, there are often osmiophilic finely granular structures of different shapes in the region of the intensely thickened internal lamina rara; this may cause obliteration of a loop. These deposits partly impress as coarse lumps (Fig. 15) which are characterized by a rather precise outline but no membrane.

Two of our cases show large osmiophilic subendothelial deposits, as can be found in lupus nephritis: case 1 with morbus Fabry, case 5 with chronic-interstitial non-destructive nephritis as primary disease (Fig. 16). 6 out of 12 patients with glomerulonephritis as primary disease showed smaller osmiophilic deposits at electron microscopy. The same applied to 4 out of 9 patients with other primary diseases (s. Table 1).

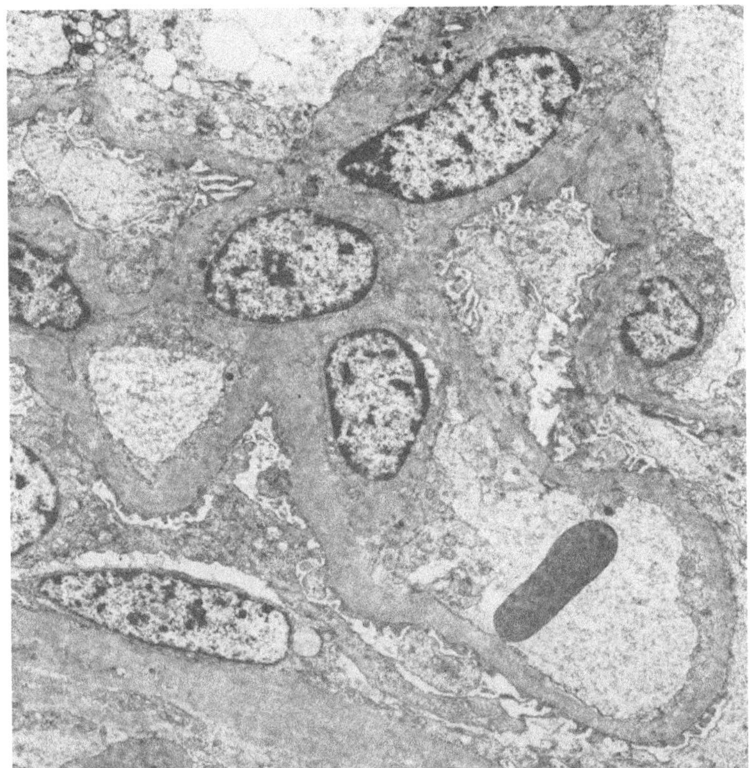

Fig. 7. Peripheral part of collapsed glomerulum, 14 months after transpl. (case 2). BM severely thickened and sporadically pleated. Mesangium not enlarged, endothelium unchanged. 3910 ×

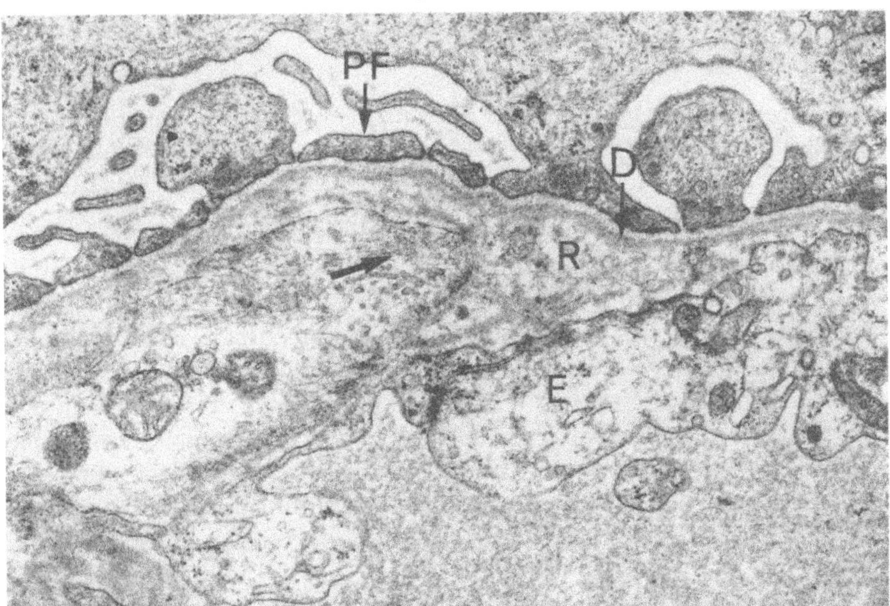

Fig. 8. Section of glomerular loop wall, 7 months after transpl. (case 20). BM as a whole thickened, lamina densa (D) rarified, lamina rara interna (R) electron-lucent, a mesangial cell is creeping into the lamina rara interna (→). Endothelial cells (E) activated, visceral epithelial cells with hinted pedical-fusion. 16900 ×

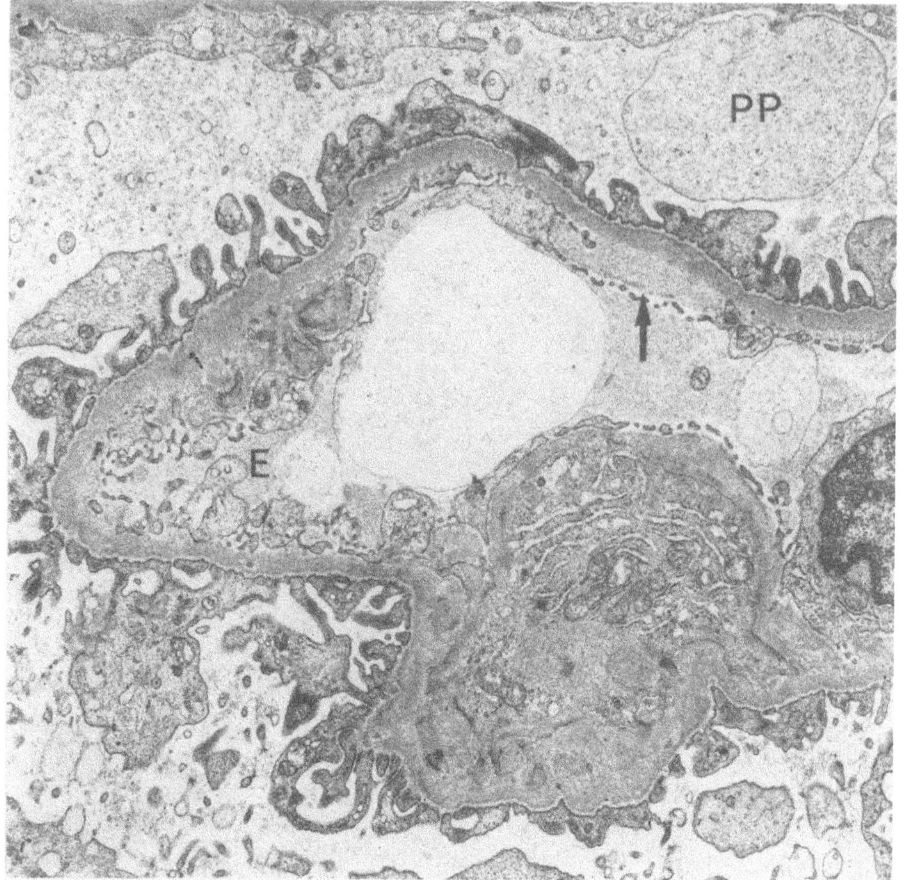

Fig. 9. Distinct TGP (+), 19 months after transpl. (case 5). Cushion-like localsized thickening of the lamina rara interna (→), endothelium with arcade formation (E), processes of visceral epithelial cells edematous (PP). Only hinted pedicular fusion. 6300 ×

Osmiophilic, narrow bands under the endothelium can be differentiated from these deposits (Fig. 17); their optic density and structure reminds of the lamina densa. From this structure all kinds of transitions lead to parallel or netlike osmiophilic layers. In some cases, an osmiophilic, rather plump fibrillar lacework developed (Fig. 17).

In the extremely severe form of TGP, light microscopy shows a clear duplication of the BM in silver-stained sections (Fig. 4). Electron microscopic studies reveal a split-up, lamina densa-like structure beneath the endothelium

Fig. 10. Very slight TGP (±), 14 months after transpl. (case 2). *R* Small electron-lucent cushion of the lamina rara interna. *PP* Edematous processe of epithelial cells. *V* Vacuoles in endothelial cells. *X* Hyaline droplet in endothelial cell. 15600 ×

Fig. 11. Nodular protrusion (*P*) on the endothelial face of the BM, 30 days after transpl. (case 6). 18000 ×

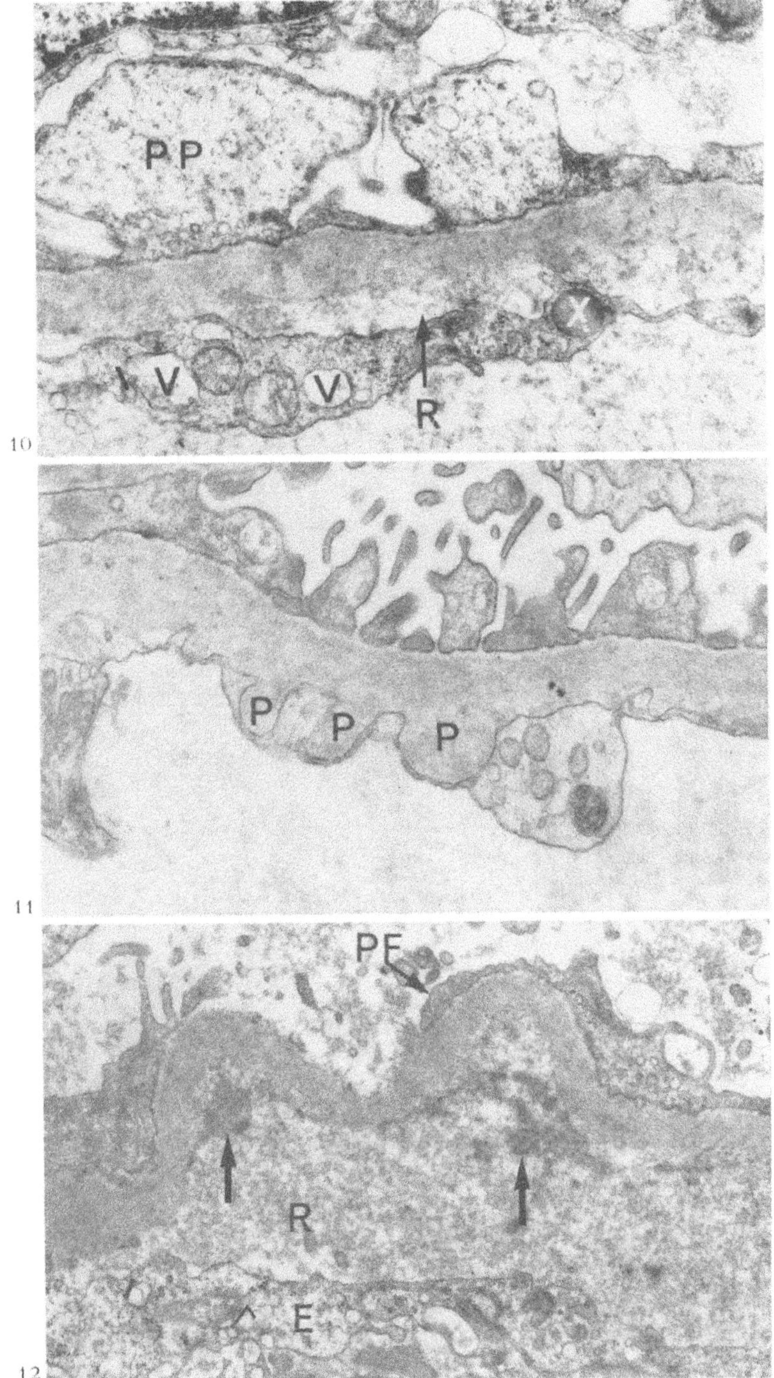

Figs. 10—12

Fig. 12. Heavy focal thickening of the lamina rara interna (*R*) in otherwise only very slight TGP, 14 months after transpl. (case 2). The finely granular, electron-lucent lamina rara interna (*R*) contains a few electron-dense, fibrillar deposits (→) (fibrin ?), the endothelium (*E*) is enlarged and vacuolar. *PF* Pedical-fusion. 12100 ×

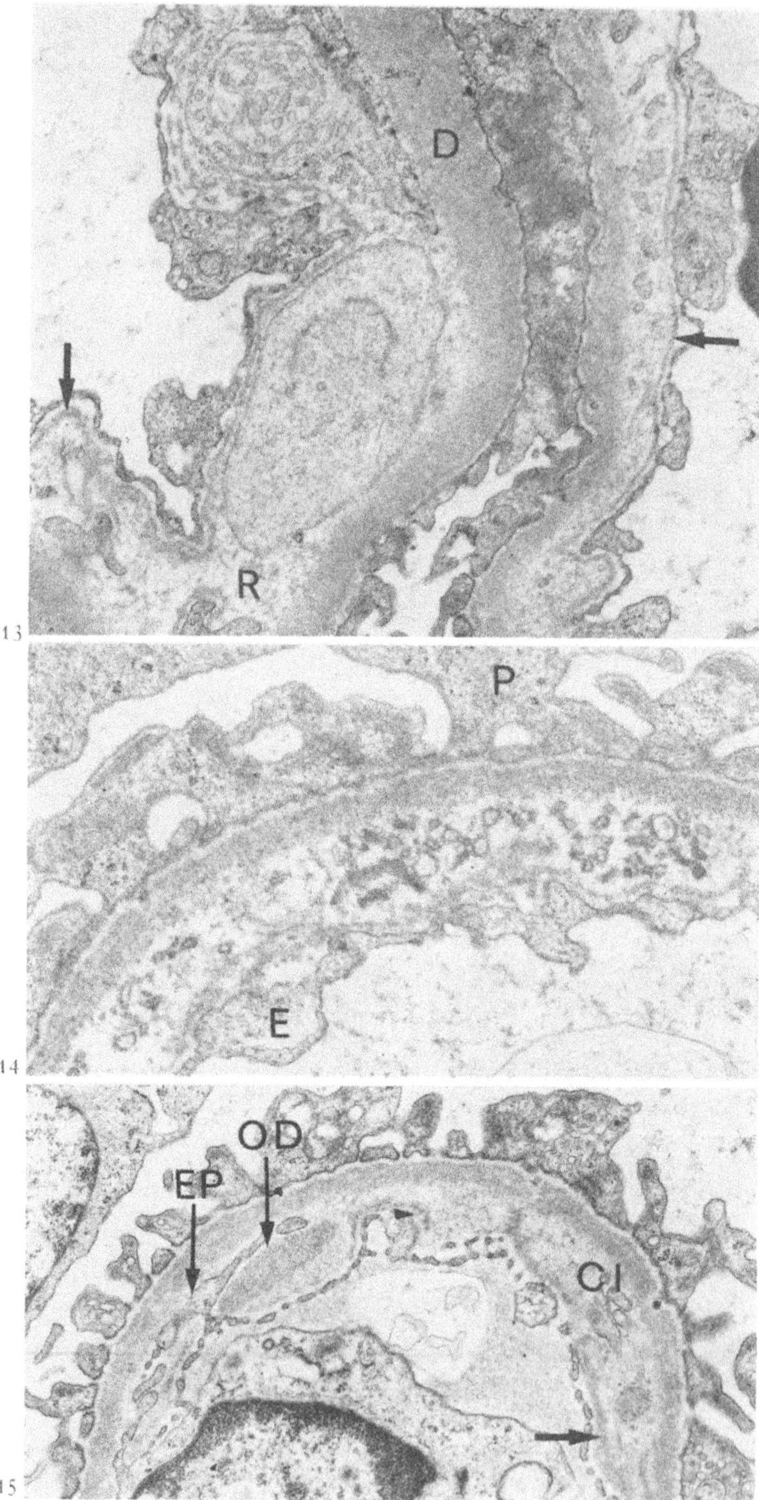

Figs. 13—15

(Figs. 8, 13, 14, 15). The enlarged loops (Fig. 19), impressing, at light microscopy, as aneurysms at first, disclose at electron microscopy a solid group of
endothelial cells in the center (Fig. 20). In extreme cases of TGP, the internal
lamina rara may measure up to 79 μ. In the finely granular masses of the
thickened internal lamina rara, only a few scattered erythrocytes can be seen

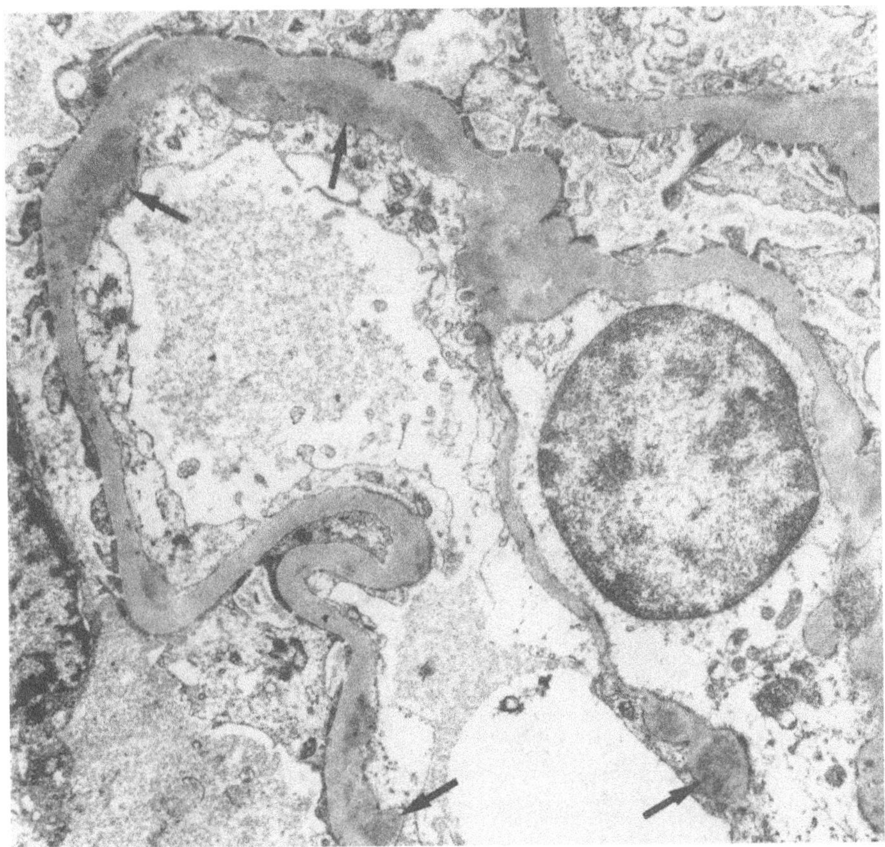

Fig. 16. Multiple osmiophilic deposits (→) on the endothelial side of the BM, 16$^1/_2$ months
after transpl. (case 1 with morbus Fabry). 4 380 ×

Fig. 13. Moderately severe TGP (+ +), 27 months after transpl. (case 8). Lamina rara
interna (*R*) grossly enlarged with enclosed cytoplasm. In both loops beneath the endothelium a thin layer of lamina densa-like substance (→). Adjoining side of lamina densa
to the lamina rara interna is not sharply defined. 11 600 ×

Fig. 14. Section of peripheral loop in TGP + +, 5$^1/_2$ months after transplant (case 13).
Multiple organelles in the grossly thickened lamina rara interna. *E* Endothelium, *P*
epithelium. 17 600 ×

Fig. 15. TGP + +, 32 months after transplant. (case 7). Heavy electron-lucent subendothelial thickening containing inclusions of cytoplasm (*CI*). Beneath the endothelium
a layer of lamina densa-like material (→). *OD* Osmiophilic deposit in the intensely thickened lamina rara interna. *EP* endothelial protrusion into lamina rara. 13 710 ×

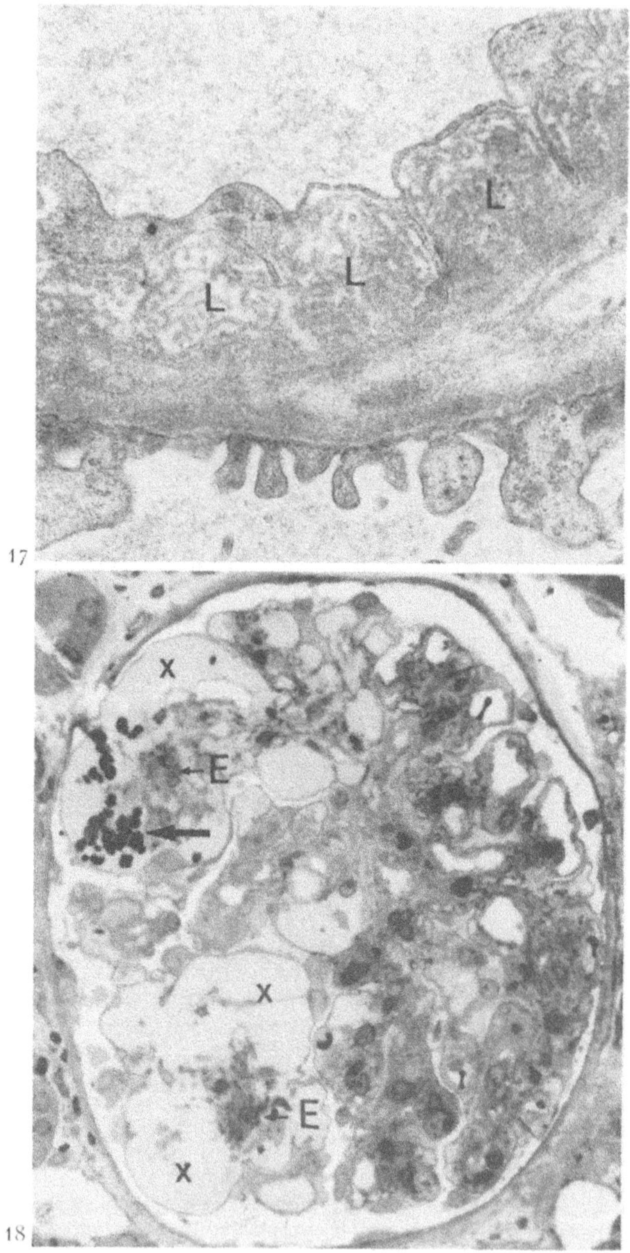

Fig. 17. Extensive lacework (*L*) of lamina densa-like structure in the intensely thickened lamina rara interna, $2^1/_2$ years after transplant. (case 11). 11 000 ×

Fig. 18. Extremely severe TGP, $2^1/_2$ years after transpl. (case 11). Two loops are grossly enlarged by an optically almost empty amorphous substance (*X*) containing some erythrocytes (→). Endothelium (*E*) compressed in the middle of the loops. Semithin section, azur eosin, 400 ×

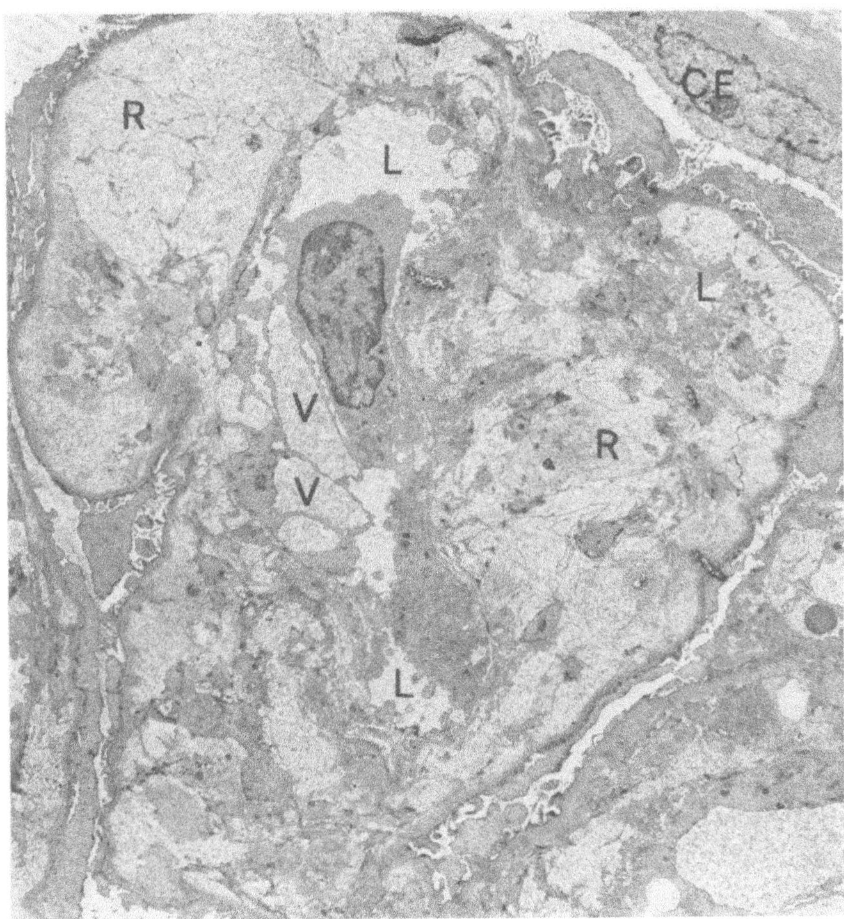

Fig. 19. Same case as Fig. 18. Two adjacent loops with extremely enlarged finely granular lamina rara interna (*R*) containing some fibrillar structures. *L* Residual caillary lumen, *V* Large vacuoles in the endothelium, *CE* Capsular epithelium. 3000 ×

(Fig. 18). Here and there, a mesangial cell is embedded (Fig. 20). In other places small vesicular structures can be observed (Fig. 14). They occur quite often in areas surrounded by membranes. These regions contain scattered mitochondria and parts of ergastoplasm. Picro-Mallory staining of semithin sections shows plenty of fibrin fibres in the thickened walls of the loops in some cases (Fig. 21). Electron microscopy revealed such fibres but in short fragments (Fig. 12, 19). This extremely severe change of the BM may sometimes lead to complete obliteration of the loops (Fig. 20); the latter, however, are ordinarily not coalesced with the glomerular capsule. Only in case 11 we found one loop completely obliterated and fused with the basement membrane of the capsule. While, as a rule, the external lamina rara of the BM seems unchanged, in one case a high-grade, irregularly nodular, mainly non-osmiophilic thickening of the subepithelial layer, i.e. of the external lamina rara,

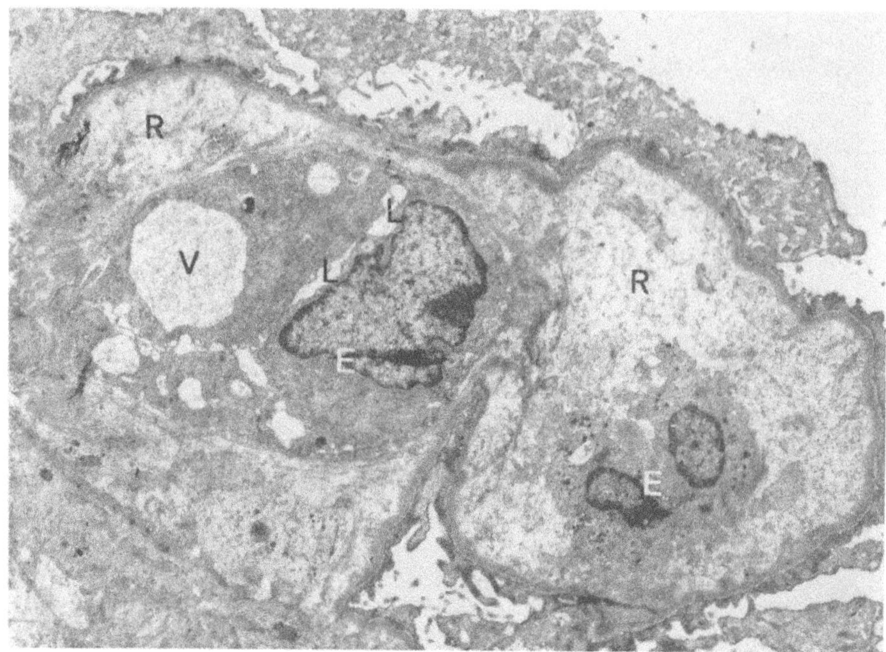

Fig. 20. Highest degree of TGP, 30 months after transplant (case 3). Electron-lucent enlargement of the lamina rara interna (R) with very fine osmiophilic graining and a few thread-like structures. Inside of lamina densa with unsharp demarkation. E Batch of endothelium without defineable lumen of the loop. L Slit-like residual lumen of amother capillary loop, its endothelial cells (E) intensely swollen, containing big vacuoles (V).
5100 ×

can be recognized (Observation 8: primary disease = diffuse glomerulo-nephritis). Only here and there, coarse osmiophilic deposits can be seen in the basement membrane, arranged alongside the mesangium (Fig. 22). Otherwise, the thickenings are of low density, finely granular, analogous to the changes of the internal lamina rara described above. Streaky osmiophilic structures are embedded again, in part running parallel to the irregularly structured basal area of the foot processes. Their density reminds of the lamina densa (Fig. 23). As a second element, larger, roundish inclusions of cytoplasm are encountered in small numbers (Fig. 24); finally, we frequently observed in rather large quantities spherular structures of approximatively 780 Å, surrounded by a membrane with dark center.

The *mesangium* shows no considerable proliferation of the nuclei; the mesangial so-called BM-like material is, however, considerably increased

Fig. 21. Severely altered singular loop of a glomerulum with very severe degree of TGP (+ + +), same case as Fig. 18 and 19. L Narrowed lumen of the loop. In the otherwise empty looking lamina rara interna multiple small fibrin threads (F). CAB, 1000 ×

Fig. 22. Subepithelial osmiophilic deposits (OD), 27 months after transplant (case 8). M Nucleus of Mesangial cell. 10200 ×

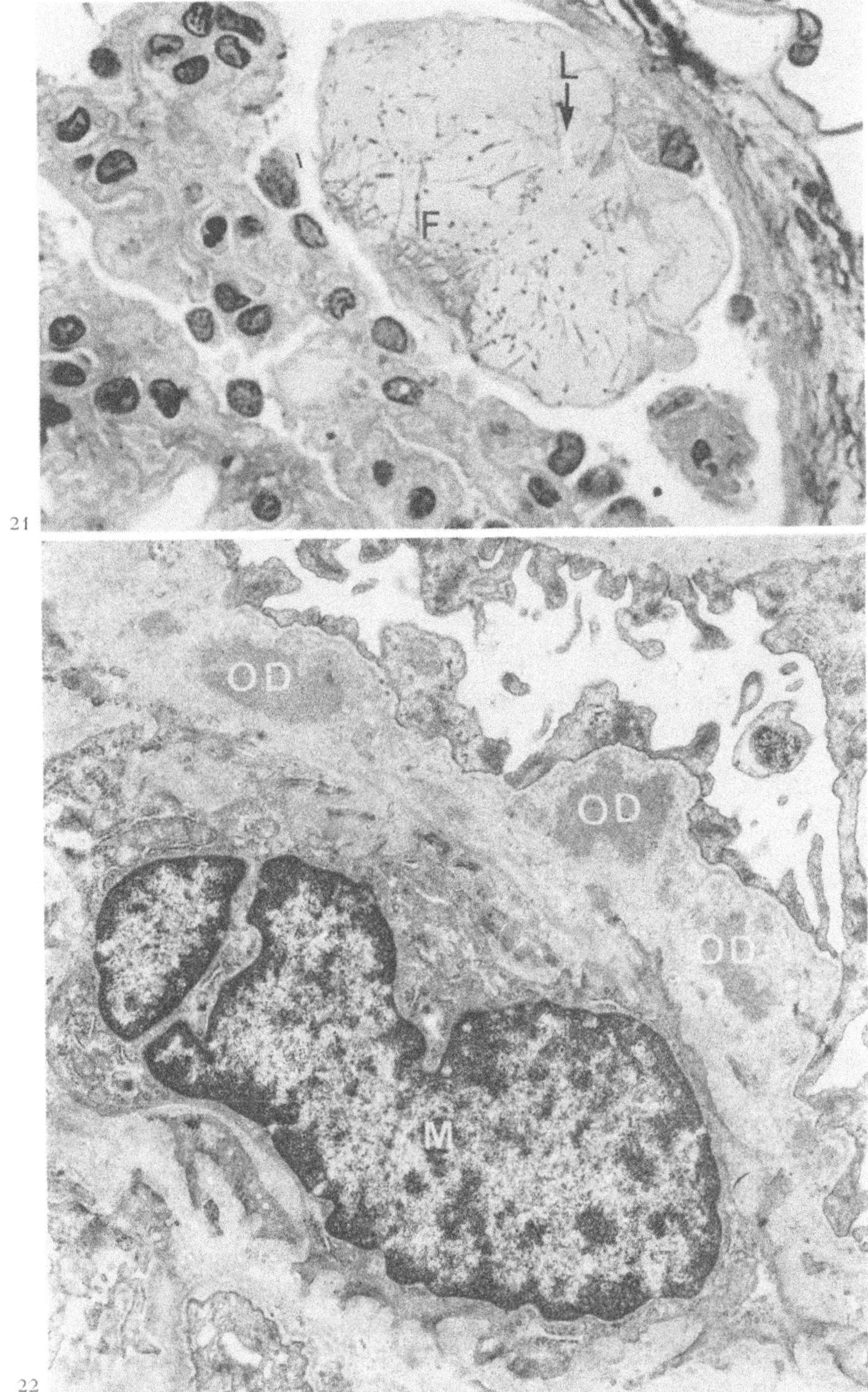

Figs. 21 and 22

2*

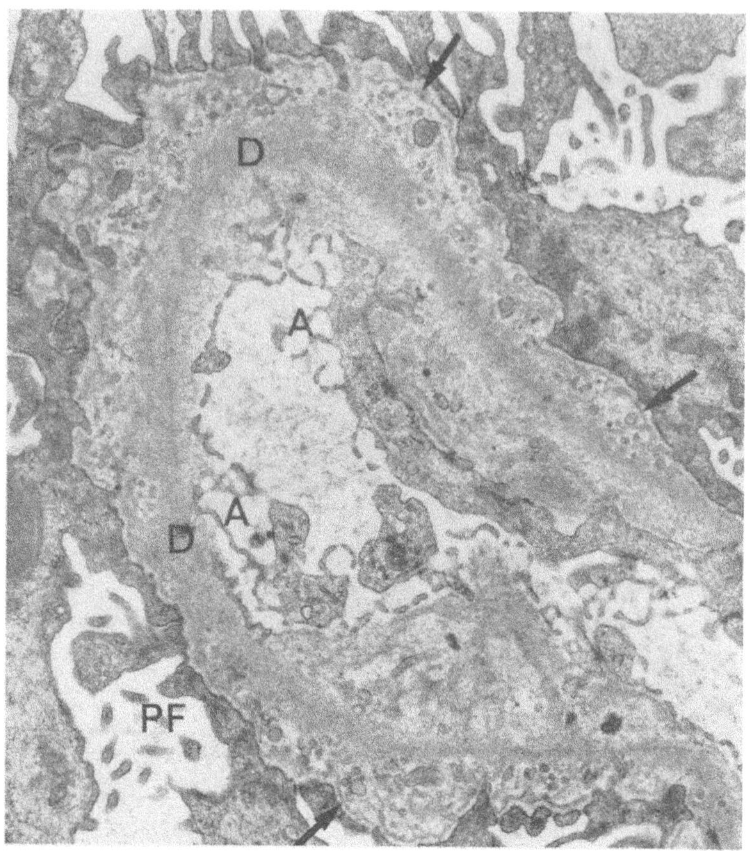

Fig. 23. Same case as Fig. 22. Lamina densa (*D*) with blurred demarkation on both sides Subendothelially electron-lucent thickening, subepithelial knot-like also electron-lucent thickenings containing spherical inclusions (s. Fig. 24). Immediately below the epithelium newly formed lamina densa (→). Arcade formation of endothelial cells (*A*). *PF* Pedical fusion. 10580 ×

(Fig. 6, 25). This BM material occasionally contains inclusions of cytoplasm, as described above. In 6 cases (5, 7, 9, 13, 14, 15) compact deposits were perceptible by light microscopy (Fig. 26); at electron microscopy, they are osmiophilic and rather precisely outlined (Fig. 27). In three cases we found foam cells in the mesangium (Fig. 28).

The *endothelial cells* are severely altered in all sections. However the damage varies from loop to loop, in quantity as well as in quality. There is, above all, a severe swelling of the endothelial cells with enlargement of the nucleus (Fig. 5). The mitochondria are unusually numerous and large, and the ergastoplasm is very prominent. Besides, the cells frequently contain vacuoles filled with material similar to that of the thickenings of the internal lamina rara (Figs. 10, 19, 20). In one case we found an endothelial foam cell (Fig. 29). The remaining lumen is often densely filled with vesicular processes or garland-shaped arcades of endothelial cell processes (Fig. 6). Two cases (1, 2) with acute rejection show thrombocytes in addition to disintegration and desquamation. One case (6) discloses several leucocytes 30 days after transplantation, and another one (14) plenty of fibrin 28 months after transplantation. Only cases with very severe TGP show complete obliteration of some loops (Fig. 30).

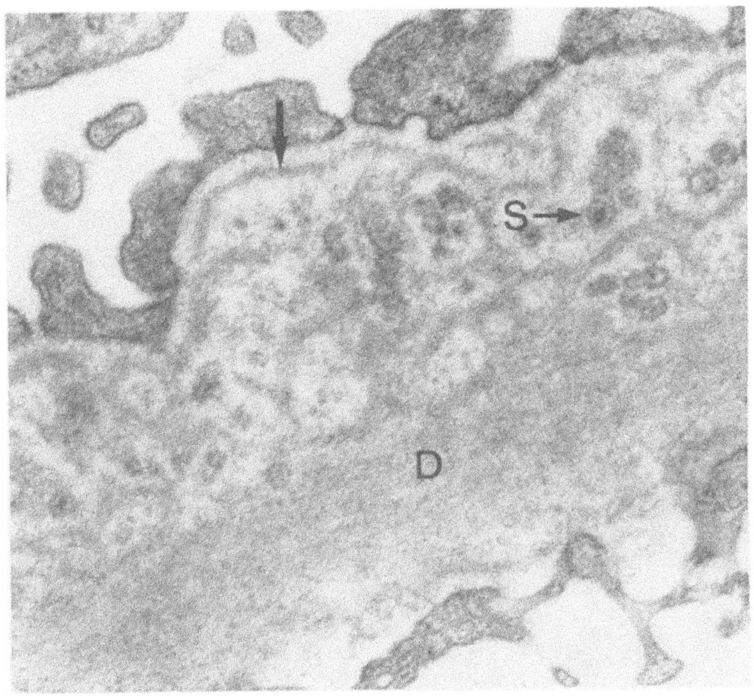

Fig. 24. Same case as Fig. 22 and 23. *S* Spherical inclusions, probably virus bodies. → Newly formed subepithelial lamina densa. *D* Original lamina densa on neither side sharply defined. 40050 ×

Usually, the alteration of the BM is especially distinct beneath the nuclear boundaries of the endothelial cells. Deposits within the endothelial cells are not present.

The *visceral epithelium cells* proliferate, as can be seen from most figures (Fig. 25 etc.). Ribosomes, the rough endoplasmic reticulum and Golgi apparatus are unusually prominent. The cells form plump processes, poor in organelles, thus being probably edematous (Fig. 25, 27). There is pedicular fusion in most cases (Fig. 6, 13, 20).

The *Bowman's capsule* is, on the whole, only slightly changed. We missed an actual proliferation of cells with the exception of case 3 (s. below). On the other hand, we found quite often hyaline droplet accumulations and myelin bodies. Cases 1, 6, 7 show homogenous osmiophilic deposits in the capsular BM. Only in one case (3) a definite, typical subacute extra- and intracapillary glomerulonephritis with proliferation of the capsular parietal epithelium

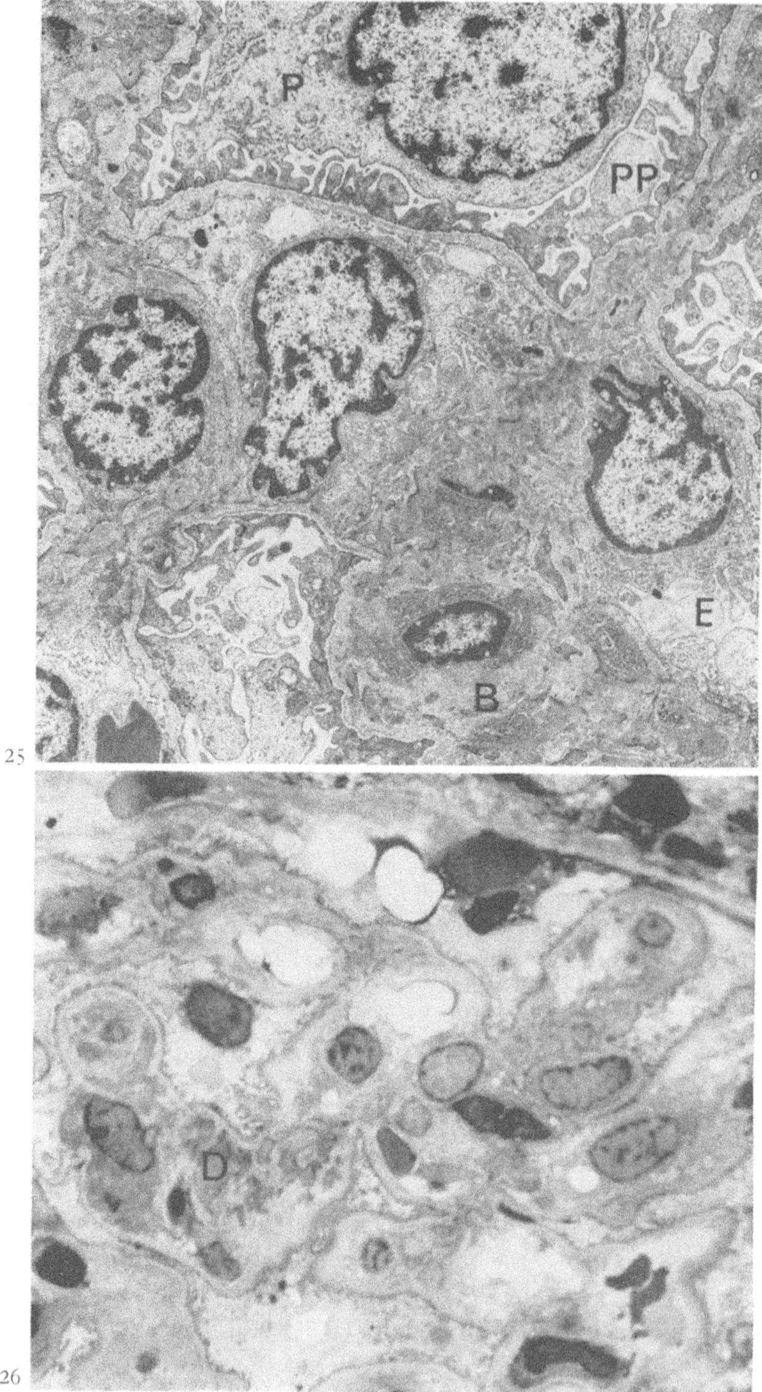

Fig. 25. Low grade TGP (+), 7 months after transplant (case 20). Distinct increase of the basement-like substance of the mesangium (*B*). Considerable swelling of the epithelial cells (*P*) and theire processes (*PP*). The same applies to the processes of the endothelium (*E*). 5130 ×

Fig. 26. Large deposits of lightoptically dense material (*D*) in moderately severe TGP (++), 5^1/$_2$ months after transplant (case 13). Semithin section, azur eosin, 1200 ×

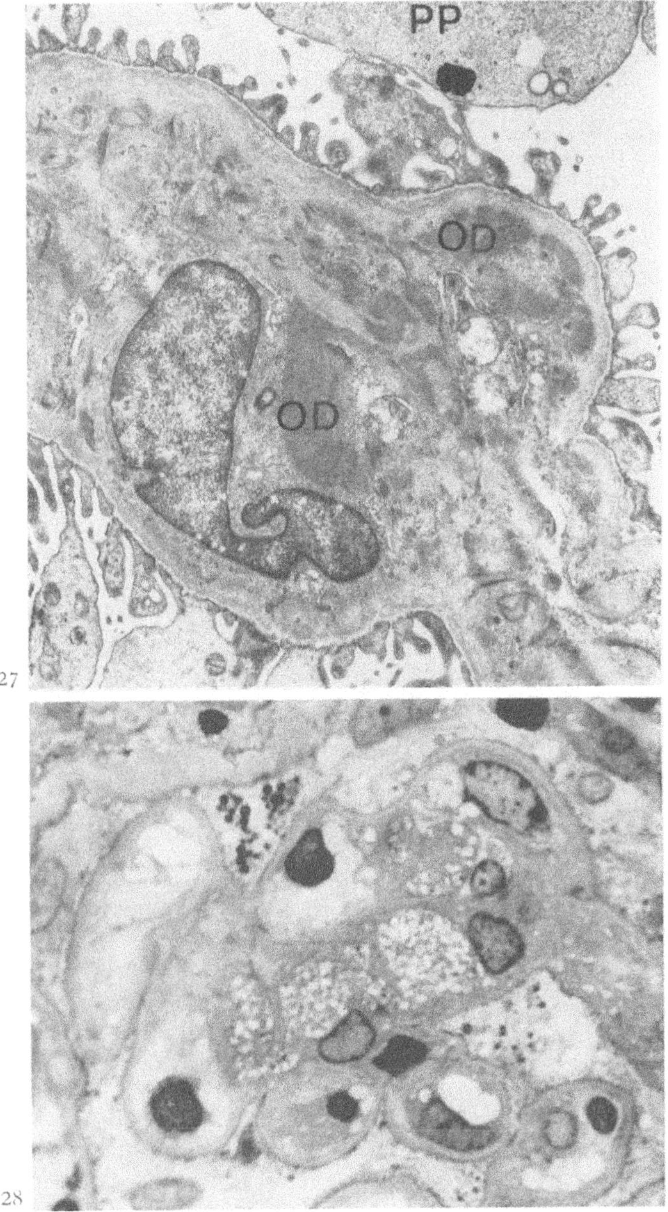

Fig. 27. Extensive mesangial osmiophilic deposits (*OD*) in moderately severe TGP (++),
32 months after transplant (case 7). 7770 ×

Fig. 28. Mesangial foam cells in TGP (++), $5^1/_2$ months after transplant. (case 13).
Semithin section, azur eosin, 1200 ×

(crescents) and beginning synechias between loops and capsule was observed.
Practically all glomerula are affected in this case. In some places, the intracapillary change has already led to obliteration of the loops (Fig. 31).

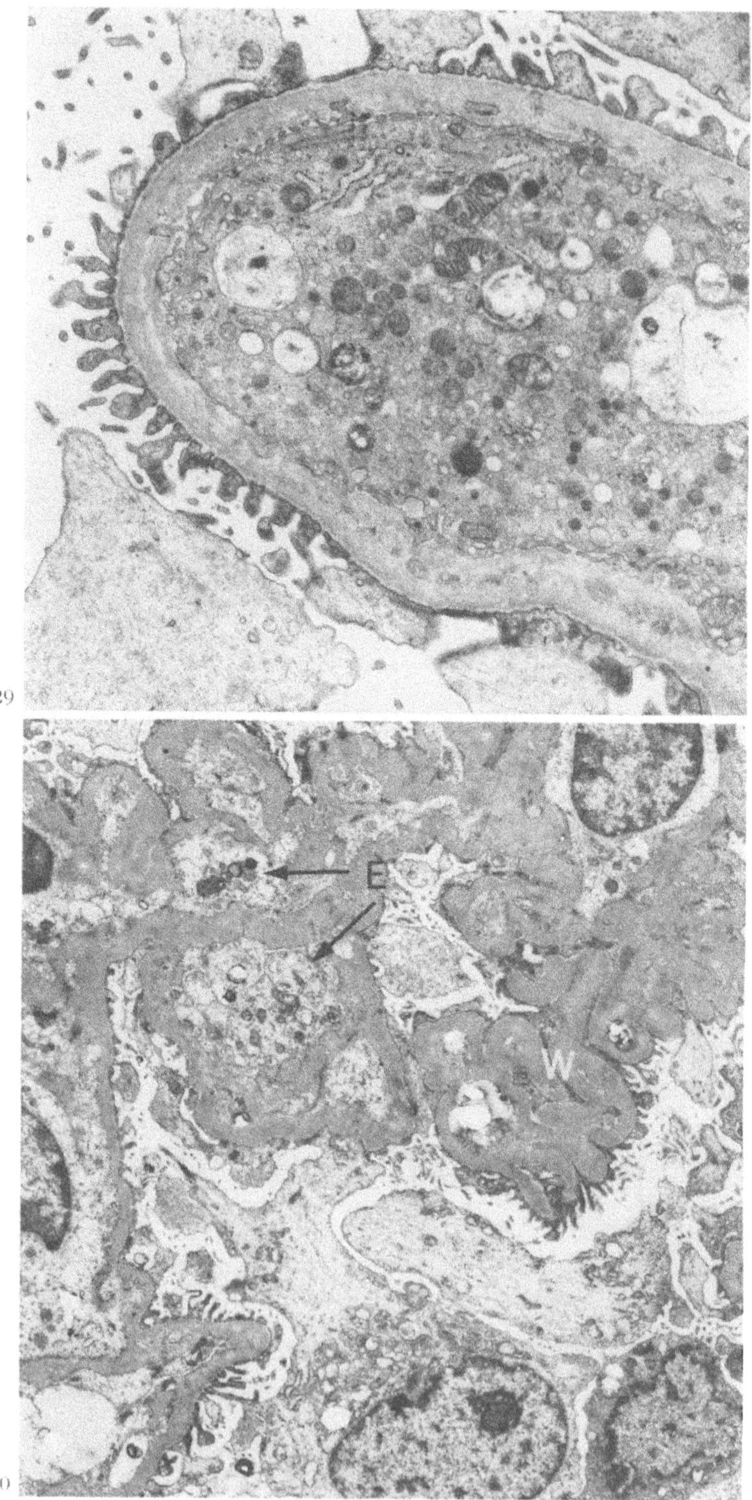

Figs. 29 and 30

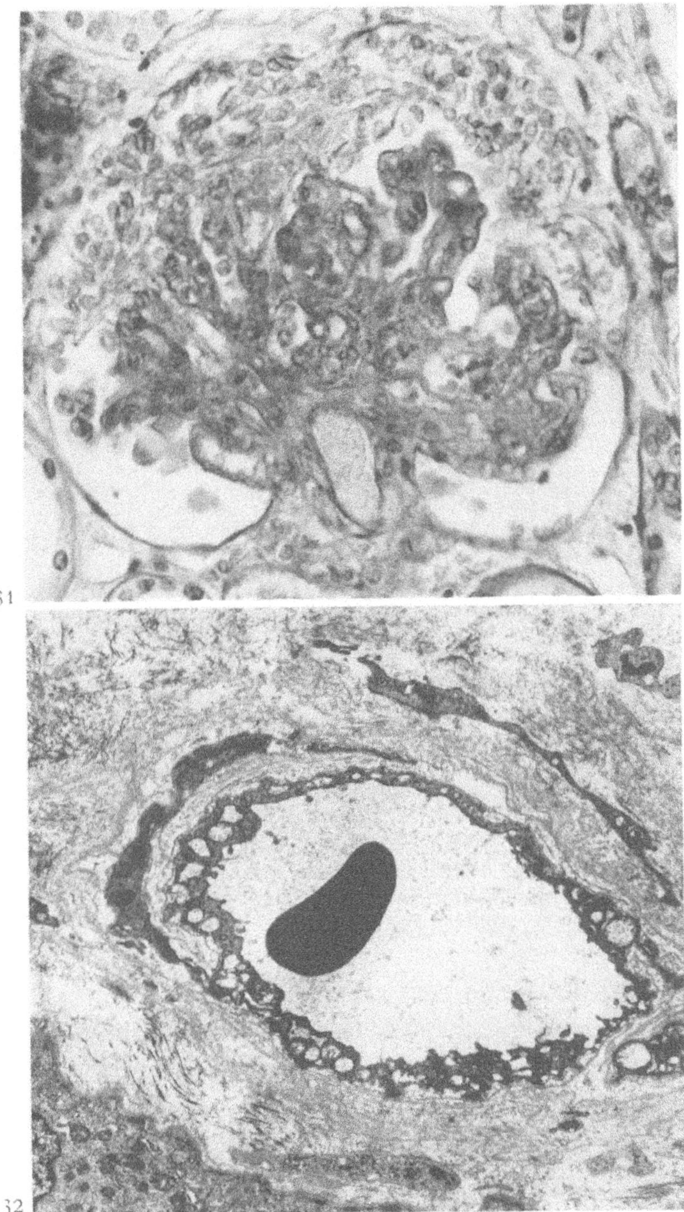

Fig. 31. Extra- and intracapillary glomerulonephritis, proliferative phase, 19 months after transplant. (case 3). Primary disease: Chronical intra- and extracapillary glomerulonephritis. PAS, 400 ×

Fig. 32. Intertubular capillary with swollen (edematous ?) endothelium containing numerous vacuoles. BM multilayered, edematously split, 3 years after transpl. (case 11). 5 180 ×

Fig. 29. Endothelial foam cell in TFP (+ +), 32 months after transpl. (case 7). BM irregularly thickened, pedicles without fusion. Pronounced edematous swelling of the epithelical all processes and of an few pedicles. 8200 ×

Fig. 30. Glomerular loops in TGP (+ + +), 23 months after transpl. (case 3). Besides the proliferation of the endothelium (E) a vascularly caused collapse of the loops recognizeable by the wrinkling of the BM (W) has lead to the devastation of the loops. 4 420 ×

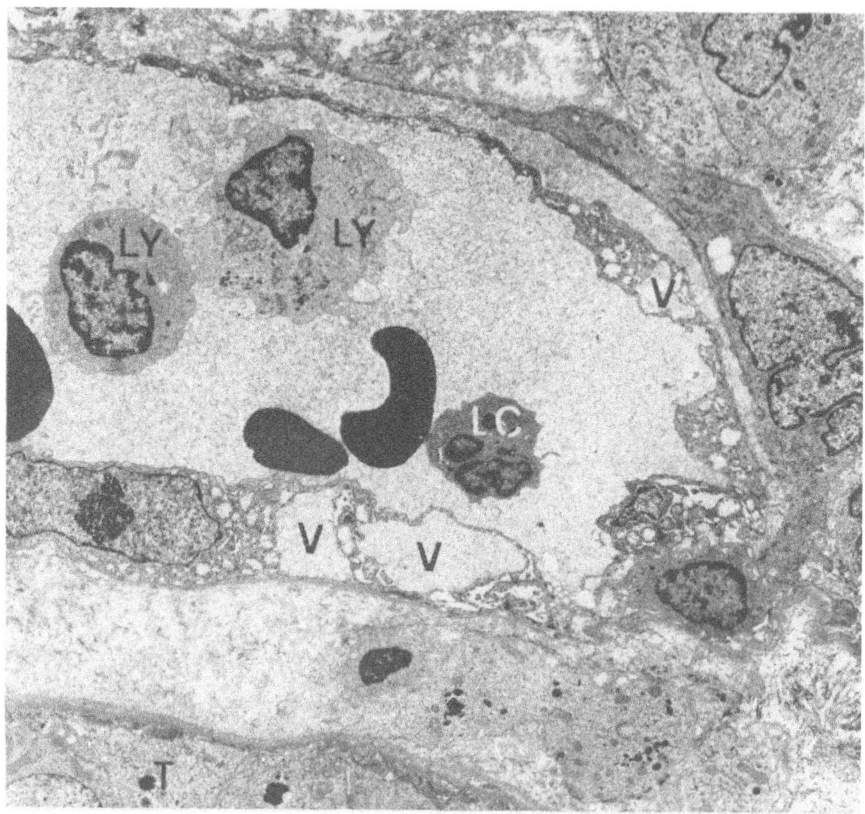

Fig. 33. Intertubular capillary, 3¹/₂ months after transpl. (case 10). Clinically no signs of rejection. In the lumen of the vessel a neutrophilic leucocyt (*LC*) and two lymphoid cells (*LY*). Endothelial cells with numerous partly very large vacuoles (*V*), *T* Adjoining tubules. Tissue between capillary and tubulus highly edematous. 3150 ×

The graphic representation of development, degree of severity of TGP, etc. (Fig. 1) makes four points clear:

1. On the average, glomerulopathy of the individual case reaches its maximum degree of severity 4–12 months after transplantation (exception: observation 8: 27 months).

2. The maxima of the individual cases vary. They range between $\pm$ and $+++$. One case (14) showed a trace of $\pm$ TGP 28 months after transplantation.

3. Once the maximum of the individual case has been reached, it seems to remain unchanged.

4. There is no interdependence between TGP and ALG therapy.

The severe changes at the inner layer of the BM and in the endothelial region made us examine the *intertubular capillaries* and look für analogous changes. This endothelium, as well as that of the loops, shows profuse proliferation with villiform projections into the lumen (Fig. 32) in almost all cases.

Here and there, fresh necrotic desquamations of the endothelium can be seen. In other cases it is possible to demonstrate grotesque formations of vacuoles (Fig. 33), similar to those of the glomerular endothelium. The BM is multiply split (Fig. 32); sometimes nodular formations are found which look quite similar to those of the glomerular capillaries. Occasionally, the BM of the arterioles has lost its compactness.

2. Immuno-Histology (s. Table 2)

In 8 patients with altogether 10 biopsies no human serum proteins were found in the area of the glomerula. In all these cases, horse ALG had been given i.v.; it could be shown by immunhistology linearly alongside the glomerular BM (Fig. 34). Morphologic examination revealed, with the exception of the third biopsy of case 6, only insignificant to slight glomerulopathies.

In the glomerula of all other biopsies, deposits of human immunoglobulins, mainly combined with C'3, were conspicuous. IgM was by far more frequently found than IgG; in many cases it was the only immunoglobin. As to the pattern of the deposits, almost all of them were granular to broken-linear, their main part always being localized in the mesangium. Usually, the changes encroached from single places of the mesangium into the periphery of the loops (Fig. 35).

As cases 7, 12, 14 and 16 show, ALG, on principle, is of no importance in the development of these deposits. Besides, no significant connection between the intensity of the immunofluorescent findings and the histologically distinct glomerulopathy was encountered.

Immunhistologic findings, indicating the host's reaction to the applied ALG, were seldom found: In 3 of the cases (1, 5, 6) a linear C'3 deposit, identical with the ALG pattern, was found once, being within the picture of a complete heterologous phase of experimental Masugi-nephritis.

In case 11 and in the third biopsy of case 10 there were findings equivalent to the autologous phase, i.e. identical patterns of ALG and the host's immunoglobulins. At the glomerular basement membranes of the latter, coarse granular deposits of ALG, immunoglobulins and complement of the host, thus a concurrent glomerulonephritis of the serum-sickness type, were additionally found. Because of identical mesangial deposits of these components a similar situation was suspected in the first biopsy of case 19. Nevertheless a morphology corresponding to the immunologic findings in the form of a genuine glomerulonephritis could not be observed in either of these cases.

3. Clinical Findings

No significant correlation could be observed between TGP and proteinuria or histocompatibility. Normal or only barely increased protein excretion (less than 600 mg/24 h) was found to be associated with severe TGP in some cases.

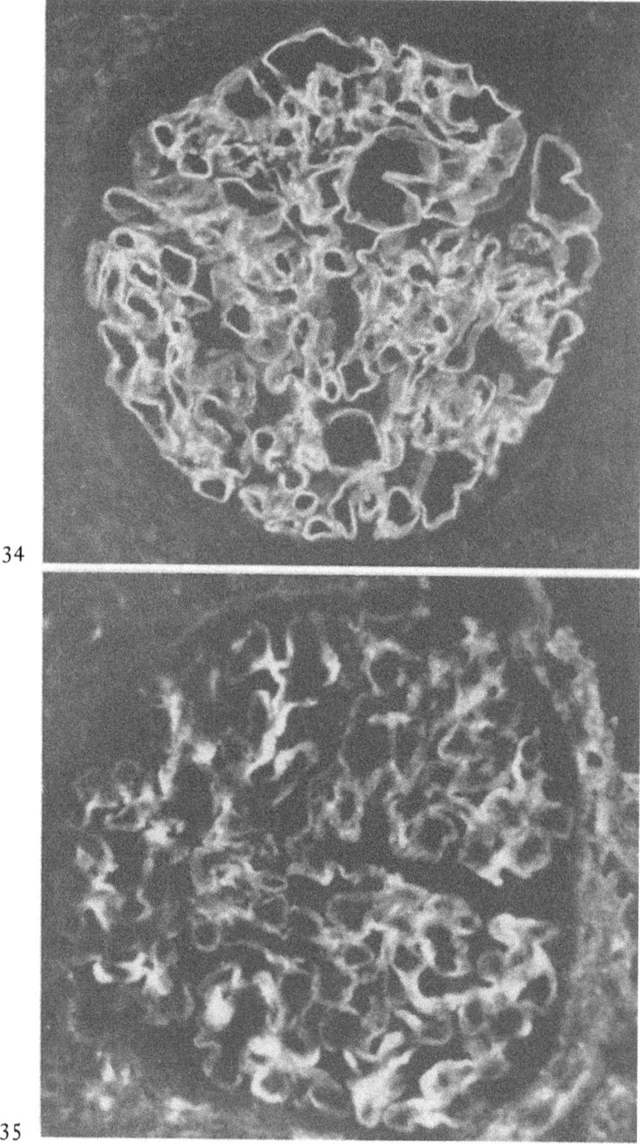

Fig. 34. Glomerulum of transplanted kidney after ALG treatment (case 15). Clear-cut linear fluorescence along the entire BM after staining for horse immunoglobulin. 360 ×

Fig. 35. Glomerulum 14 months after transpl. and ALG treatment (case 8). Immuno-fluorescent staining for human IgM. Focal finely granular deposits of IgM are present mainly within mesangial areas and in some of the capillary walls. An analogous pattern was seen after staining for human β 1 C/1 A. 330 ×

On the other hand, some patients with minimum glomerular changes were excreting more than 1.0 g (Fig. 36). In general, proteinuria tended to increase 6 months after transplantation but again, constant or increasing proteinuria

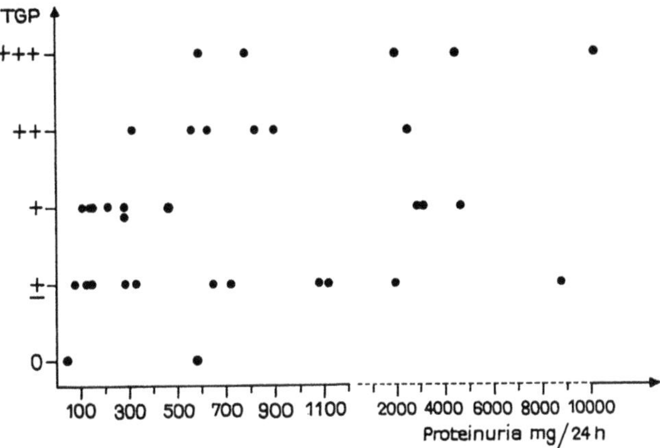

Fig. 36. Correlation between TGP and proteinuria at the time of histologic examination. No correlation can be found. Both, minimal ($\pm$) or severe ($+++$) TGP can go along with heavy or mild proteinuria. Protein excretion below 700 mg/d does not necessarily exclude the presence of even severe TGP

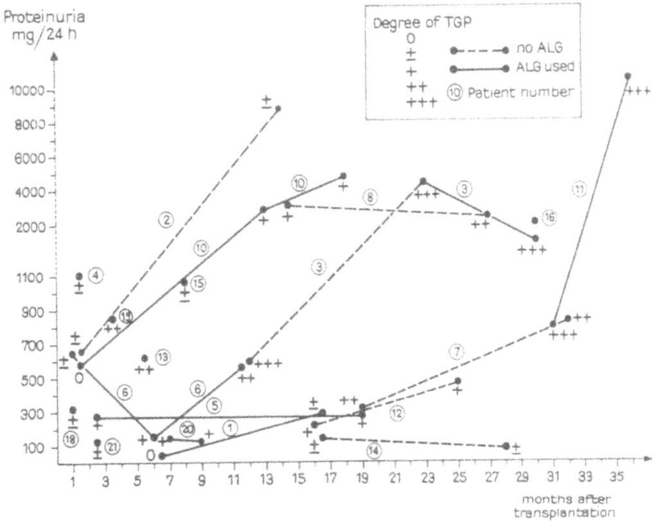

Fig. 37. Follow-up of proteinuria and TGP with time after transpl. A line of communication is drawn if several histologic examinations were performed in a single patient. There is a general trend of proteinuria to increase after 6 months. Comparing the development of TGP and proteinuria a non-parallel behavior can be seen in several patients (cases 2, 3, 8 and 11). Patients with and without ALG show a similar pattern and scatter of proteinuria. Note: all ALG was given intravenously and contained always anti-glomerular-basement-membrane antibodies

was not necessarily associated with a parallel behaviour of TGP (Fig. 37). Comparing the creatine clearance with degrees of TGP (Fig. 38), the mean clearance was significantly higher in grafts with slight ($+$) compared to those

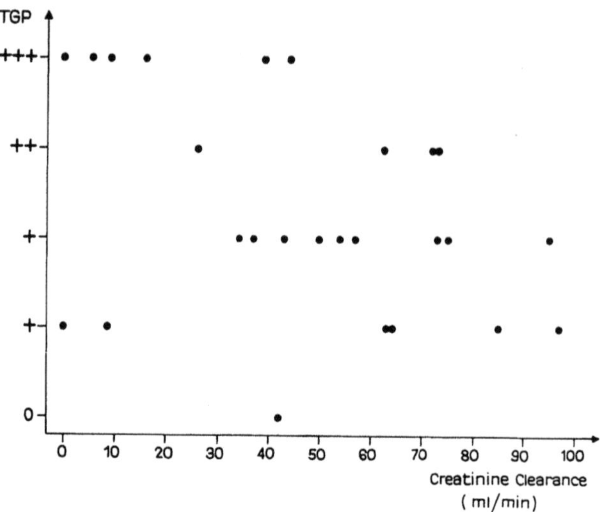

Fig. 38. Creatinine clearance and TGP show some correlation if only examinations after a minimal post-transplant follow-up of 6 months were considered. Allografts with severe TGP (+++) have a creatinine clearance of 19 ± 18 ml/min (mean and SD). Kidneys with mild TGP (+) have a significantly higher creatinine clearance of 58 ± 20 ml/min ($p < 0.005$)

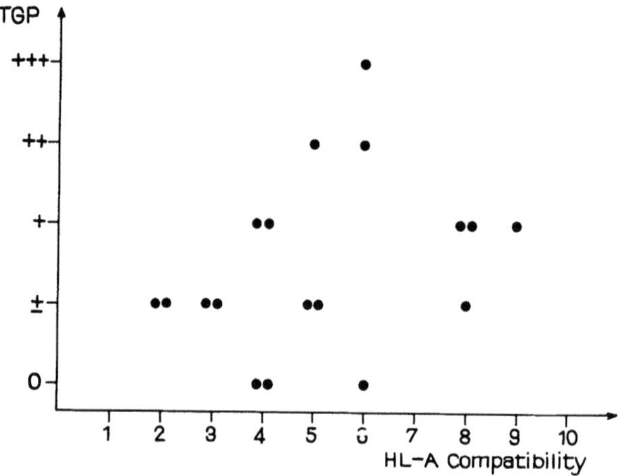

Fig. 39. Comparing HL-A-compatibility (ranking of Rappaport and Dausset) with TGP there is some trend of TGP to get worse with increasing incompatibility. However, the scatter is too big to reach any level of significance

with severe TGP (+++) (19 ± 18 ml/min versus 58 ± 20 ml/min) (p 0.005). Histocompatibility expressed with HL-A-compatibility ranking (Fig. 39), or number of rejection episodes (Fig. 40) or an overall Clinical Compatibility Classification (Fig. 41), as defined in chapter Material and Methods, showed in each instance a trend to decrease with increasing TGP. However, the scatter was far too wide to draw any definite conclusion.

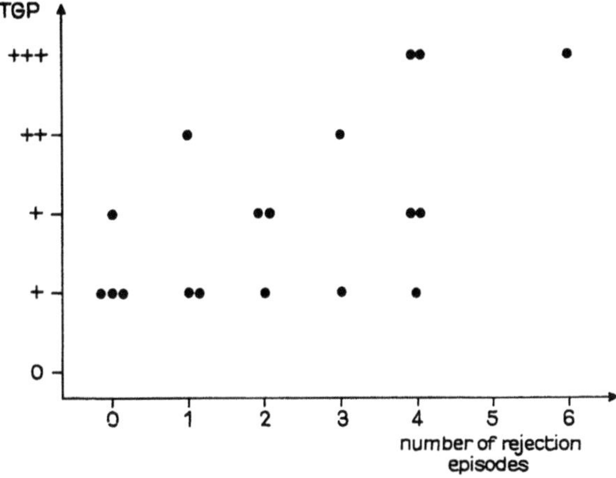

Fig. 40. The number of acute rejection episodes correlates poorly with the degree of TGP. Despite much scatter some trend seems visible however. Minimal TGP was found in 5 out of 7 patients with not more than one rejection episode, compared to 1 out of 6 patients with four or more rejection crises

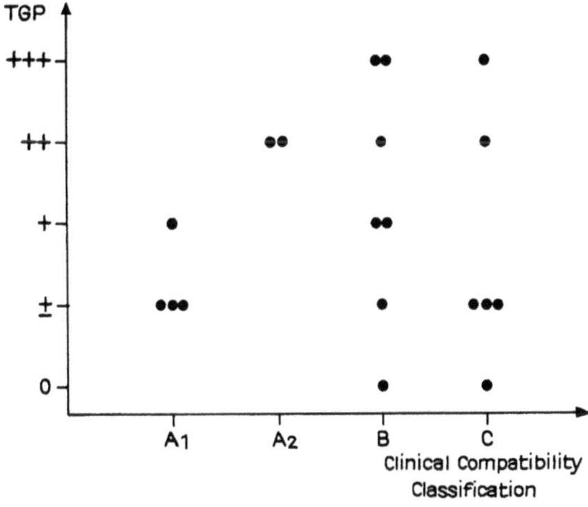

Fig. 41. The overall clinical compatibility classification (defined in chapter on material and methods) shows no clear correlation with TGP. Patients with allografts proven to be incompatible by the clinical follow-up (B and C) can show all degrees of TGP. The only distinct group is formed by those patients with a perfect course and no clinical signs of rejection (A_1). Here only minimal ($\pm$) or mild ($+$) TGP is found

C. Discussion

Only glomerular changes, whose inflammatory nature cannot be proven by structural changes, were identified as chronic transplant glomerulopathy (TGP). TGP is frequent; we were able to find it in all but one transplants which survived for more than $1^1/_2$ months (LINDQUIST *et al.*, 1968: 50%, BUSCH *et al.*, 1971a: 9/14). Only severe degrees of TGP can be recognized by light microscopy. In these cases, it reminds of a membranous glomerulonephritis for which it was occasionally mistaken (KRIEG *et al.*, 1960).

Electron microscopy reveals a thickening of the basement membrane (BM) of the glomerular loops, caused by enlargement of the internal lamina rara (Rosenau et al., 1969; Fish et al., 1967; Weymouth et al., 1970; Hume et al., 1970; Starzl et al., 1967b; Iwasaki et al., 1967 (dogs); Lindquist et al., 1969b (rats). To confound it with glomerular collapse becomes thus impossible, for in the latter, mainly the lamina densa is enlarged, and the entire BM is undulated. In extremely severe cases of TGP, the thickened internal lamina rara alone measures up to 200 times (79 μ) the diameter of the normal BM (Fig. 21; Busch et al., 1971a: 4 μ). It may contain fibrin fibrilles (see Busch et al., 1971a) and is often designated as "deposition" (Iwasaki et al., 1967; Porter et al., 1967; Glassock et al., 1968, Hamburger et al., 1966; Lindquist et al., 1970 a. o). In the thickened internal lamina rara single cell organelles and cell fragments respectively (Hume et al., 170: 50%) or whole cells of mesangial or endothelial nature can be identified (Porter et al., 1967). In our material, the change is conspicuous for the first time $1^1/_2$ months after transplantation; after 9–12 months it seems to have reached its maximum and to remain then stable (Fig. 1).

The finely granular thickening of the internal lamina rara does not seem to be reversible (cf. also Fries et al., 1970). Some authors attribute this change to ALG medication (Iwasaki et al., 1967: dogs, Lindquist et al., 1969b: rats, Hume et al., 1970; Starzl et al., 1967b: man).

We interpret the rather dense, band-like structures beneath the endothelium as a replication of the BM by newly formed lamina densa material. Its structure appears very irregular and lace-like (Fig. 17). The result is a duplication of the BM, mainly conspicuous in silver-stained semi-thin sections (Fig. 4) (cf. also Andres et al., 1970; Fish et al., 1966; Rowland et al., 1970; Busch et al., 1971a). A similar duplication of the BM is also occasionally found in chronic glomerulonephritis (Simon and Chatelanat, 1969; Strunk et al., 1964; McManus and Lupton, 1966; Churg and Grishham, 1969; Arakawa and Kimmelstiel, 1968; Ehrenreich and Churg, 1968; Bariéty et al., 1968, 1969; a.o.), though chronic glomerulonephritis lacks the finely granular, loose deposits between the layers.

The authors generally agree on the BM being principally formed by visceral epithelium. Slight participation of the endothelium in the formation of the membrane in transplant glomerulopathy seems probable; it has been assumed in other affections as well (Andres et al., 1970; Simon and Chatelanat, 1969; McManus and Lupton, 1966; Strunk et al., 1964; Madrazo et al., 1969, 1970; Rosen et al., 1968). According to Rouiller (1969) and Fish et al. (1967) the formation of a double membrane results, if the removal of resorbed material is help up.

Six times, twice in consecutive biopsies (cf. also Porter et al., 1967; Rowland et al., 1970; Fries et al., 1970), we found *subendothelial, osmiophilic deposits*, possibly equal to those of the experimental Masugi type of glomerulonephritis. They are often irregularly nodular, appearing as well without ALG therapy (Traeger et al., 1969) as in cases without primary glomerulonephritis (cf. also HAMBURGER and DORMONT, 1968). Like the finely granular thickening of the internal lamina rara (FRIES *et al.*, 1970), the osmiophilic subendothelial deposits do not seem to disappear in transplants later on.

Subepithelial osmiophilic deposits, which would be equal to the immuno-complex type of nephritis, can be seen in some cases (BUSCH *et al.*, 1971a). They were described by PORTER *et al.* (1967/68). WILLIAMS *et al.* (1968) and GLASSOCK *et al.* (1968) in the shape of so-called humps, however only in relapses of glomerulonephritis. They are also found in mice and dogs, ostensibly after ALG medication (COHEN *et al.*, 1970; HUME *et al.*, 1970, lit.). Our material lacked such osmiophilic deposits in all cases. Only in one patient (8) irregular, pale deposits with spherical, sharply outlined bodies were found subepithelially, which may be interpreted as viruses; these formations have no similiarity to humps.

In our opinion, the osmiophilic deposits — wherever they are located — are possibly the result of the formation of immunologic complexes or rather of the formation of reaction products. They do not prove the immunologic nature of the disease and do not seem to be an integrating element of TGP.

The nodular *subepithelial formations* of our observation 8 after $14^1/_2$ months and 27 months respectively, are really something special. A similar change was described by ROWLANDS *et al.* (1970) and by BUSCH *et al.* (1971a). These author's figures also show virus-suspicious spherical particles like our case 8. In our case, the serologic virus identification could not be furnished as yet.

An enlargement of the *mesangium* with increased formation of basement-like material is, especially in the late phase, described by nearly all authors and is usually interpreted as proliferation (FISH *et al.*, 1967; LINDQUIST *et al.*, 1969 and 1970; FRIES *et al.*, 1970; STARZL *et al.*, 1967b, 1968; IWASAKI *et al.*, 1967; RUSSELL, 1968; ROSSMANN *et al.*, 1969; PORTER *et al.*, 1967; BUSCH *et al.*, 1971a). We did not find profuse multiplication of the nuclei and observed mild multiplication only in extremely severe cases of TGP. The increased basement membrane-like material is, in our opinion, non-specific; it is in-creasingly formed by the mesangial cells in different diseases (McMANUS and LUPTON, 1966; PIERCE and NAKANE, 1969). The sideways insertion of mesangial cell processes under the endothelium (IRINO and HAMAMOTO, 1966; FAITH and TRUMP, 1966; ANDRES *et al.*, 1970; STARZL *et al.*, 1967b), as occasionally observed in glomerulonephritis, could be disclosed by us but in traces. The endothelial cells penetrate the BM (PORTER *et al.*, 1967) only in a few cases. Mesangial foam cells, we observed in 3 of our cases (general lit. see ZOLLINGER and ROHR, 1969), have not been described in TGP until now. Endothelial foam cells are very well known, though in transplant arteriopathy. In part, they have been interpreted as caused by disintegration of thrombocytes (PORTER *et al.*, 1964a, 1963). — Osmiophilic mesangial deposits were identified only 6 times (cf. also FISH *et al.*, 1966; PORTER *et al.*; 1967).

In acute rejection, damage of the *glomerular endothelium* is very important. In recovery, endothelium is newly formed (PORTER *et al.*, 1967; PETERSON *et al.*, 1966). In the region of the intertubular capillaries this change is generally thought to be the earliest symptom in acute rejection (Peterson *et al.*, 1966; Harlan *et al.*, 1967; Hamburger *et al.*, 1966/68; Crosnier, 1969). In chronic transplant glomerulopathy, a severe hypertrophy of the endothelium is found in some cases. Besides a distinct proliferation with formation of arcades is observed (Hume *et al.*, 1970; Fish *et al.*, 1967; Hamburger *et al.*, 1967; Lindquist *et al.*, 1968/71. Rossmann *et al.*, 1969). The swelling of the cells may partly lead to obstruction of the lumen (Starzl *et al.*, 1967b). The endothelial vacuoles containing finely granular material, electron optically similar to that of the modified internal lamina rara, seem to indicate a disturbance of the

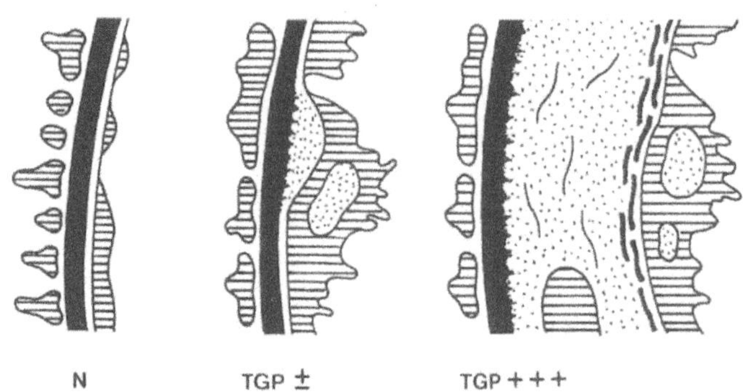

Fig. 42. Schematic representation of the alterations in the peripheral capillary loop in TGP. *n* Normal wall of loop. On the left foot processes. Black: lamina densa of BM. Narrow lamina rara interna between densa and endothelium (on the right). *G* ± Very slight TGP. Electron-lucent thickening of the lamina rara interna in a circumscript area with osmiophilic granula. Proliferative alteration of the endothelium with numerous villous processes. *G* + + + Severest degree of TGP. Lamina rara interna extremely enlarged and electron-lucent. Besides the osmiophilic granules enclosures of cytoplasm are to be found. Furthermore this area contains occasional fibrin threads and below the endothelium newly formed fragments of lamina densa. The original lamina densa shows a blurred demarkation on its endothelial face

endothelial transport mechanism. Altogether the alteration of the endothelial cells is by far the most eye-catching of all *cellular* changes in chronic TGP! For a synopsis of the main changes of the glomular wall in TGP see Fig. 42.

Activation of visceral epithelial cells varies, formation of numerous fine cellular processes is frequent. This change, however, is nonspecific; it has been observed in numerous diseases leading to severe chronic proteinuria. It may be a matter of a non-specific secondary reaction to the increased permeability of the loops. Fusion of the podocytic pedicles is often found; however not regularly in TGP (Busch *et al.*, 1971a: 100%).

Whereas we found the capsular epithelium to be only slightly changed, we discovered osmiophilic deposits in the capsular basement membrane in 3 cases. Since they can occasionally be found in pyelonephritides and other diseases of the kidney as well, we tend to interpret them as non-specific.

Genuine synechias of the loops and capsule existed only in one observation (3), but there in considerable numbers. This observation is unique in our series and is in opposition to the statements of PORTER *et al.* (1967): 37% of the cases, as well as of IWASAKI *et al.* (1967) and HUME *et al.* (1970).

Fig. 1 informs about the course of the glomerulopathy and the correlation between degree of severity, therapy and length of time. The graphic representation shows that the cases reach various degrees of severity, that the individual maximum is reached after 4–12 months (exception: case 8), that there is no relation to ALG therapy, and that the change, at least during the period of our observations (max. 36 months), shows no proneness to restitution. An observation carried out aside from the described series (pcte 694) made an extremely severe TGP even 6 weeks after transplantation conspicuous. In this case, however, any therapy had been discontinued one month before puncture and kidney removal, as kidney function was nil and hemodialysis had become necessary.

Two categories of problems are recognized by the *immunohistological findings:* On the one hand, glomerular changes are observed independently of an ALG therapy; on the other, deposits of horse gammaglobulin appearing partly in combination with an immune response of the host.

Typical of the first group are granular to broken-linear, mainly mesangial deposits of immunoglobuline and complement. We encounter the broken-linear deposits far more frequently than the purely granular ones (cf. also FISH *et al.*, 1966, 1967; LINDQUIST *et al.*, 1968; HUME *et al.*, 1970; TRAEGER *et al.*, 1969 (2 out of 15 cases), FRIES *et al.*, 1970). As these deposits are focal, deposition of circulating antigen antibody complexes is, with reference to the experimental glomerulonephritis of the serum-sickness type, discussed by some authors (LINDQUIST *et al.*, 1968; ANDRES *et al.*, 1970). The participation of transplant antigens reaching circulation has repeatedly been considered (e. g. ANDRES *et al.*, 1970), but not been proven in humans. Recently, the broken-bodies against HL-A antigens fixed on the surface of glomerular, particularly endothelial cells (BUSCH *et al.*, 1971 a).

On sole grounds of immunohistology, a glomerulonephritis of the complex type cannot be excluded in these cases with certainty, although IgG-containing deposits are said to prevail (GLASSOCK *et al.*, 1968).

The prevalence of IgM as against IgG-deposits we observed was also described by PORTER *et al.* (1968) (cf. also BUSCH *et al.*, 1968; STARZL *et al.*, 1967b; FRIES *et al.*, 1970; McPHAUL *et al.*, 1970: 6 out of 19 cases, TRAEGER *et al.*, 1969: 5 out of 15 cases), though according to CROSNIER (1969) IgG is said to be more frequent than IgM. In explanation of this phenomenon a prevailing restriction of the IgG synthesis under azathioprine is discussed (STOCKER *et al.*, 1969). KANO and MILGROM (1969) however suppose it to be an IgM antibody similar to the rheumatoid factor concealing primary IgG deposits in the glomerula.

In 12 out of 32 immunohistologically examined specimens we could identify fibrin resp. fibrinogen, twice in the lumina of the loops (cf. also ANDRES *et al.*,

1970), in the other cases as frequently mesangially as in the periphery of the loops. According to some authors, fibrin is said to exist to a higher amount in the mesangium (Lindquist *et al.*, 1968a, b; Hume *et al.*, 1970). Fries *et al.* (1970) could find neither fibrin nor complement in their cases.

Comparing expansion and intensity of the immunohistologic findings with the morphologic changes in this group, we could, like other authors (Lindquist *et al.*, 1968; Rosenau *et al.*, 1969; Busch *et al.*, 1971a), find no clear correlation. Electron microscopy reveals cases with large osmiophilic deposits. Immunofluorescence however is negative with regard to the mesangium (9). Other cases show positive mesangial immunofluorescence, but no electron microscopic deposits in this area. In agreement with the other authors, there is, consequently, no specific pattern of deposits that exists in TGP alone. A few immunofluorescent findings vary slightly from one examination to the other (3, 10, 11, 5); others, however (e.g. case 7), stay the same over a very long period of time.

Our observations disclosed minimum or lacking immunofluorescence in extremely severe glomerulopathy and highly enlarged internal lamina rara. Usually, the enlarged areas were IF-negative! Consequently, we must surmise that plasma proteins are deposited in the thickened internal lamina rara without the existence of an immune reaction, as this can be made probable by electron microscopy.

We found horse gammaglobulin as a linear layer along the glomerular basement membrane in all but one (case 8: biopsy 14 months after 40 ml ALG) cases treated with ALG. The pattern of the deposits was identical with the immunohistologic picture of the experimental Masugi nephritis and made a contamination of the used ALG with antibodies against the BM likely. The ALG was derived from horses which had been immunized by suspensions rich in cells of lymphatic organs (spleen, lymph nodes). Thus, the formation of antibodies against non-cellular structures, like reticular fibres and BM, was possible. In Rhesus monkeys, a severe nephrotoxic glomerulonephritis could be induced by large doses of our ALG (Moppert *et al.*, 1970; Thiel *et al.*, 1971). Besides, we could identify immunohistologically (case 1 and 3) horse gammaglobulin not only in the glomerula but also in the reticular framework of the spleen of two patients (Moppert *et al.*, 1970). Thus, the assumption that the used ALG contained antibodies against an antigen common to the glomerular BM and the reticular framework of lymphatic organs seems justified (cf. also Orr *et al.*, 1970). Nevertheless, anti-BM antibodies may develop even after immunization with pure lymphocytes (Busch *et al.*, 1971b).

As a rule, these nephrotoxic antibodies seem to reach the glomerula only after intravenous application: After intramuscular injection, Traeger *et al.*, (1969) and Starzl *et al.* (1967b) could not find any ALG in transplant biopsies of their patients. In the literature, Hume *et al.* (1970) came across only one case out of 40 cases with positive horse gammaglobulin identification. Busch *et al.* (1971b) reported on two cases in a series of 32 ALG-treated hosts with homografts.

In animal experiments [IWASAKI *et al.*, 1967: dogs; LINDQUIST *et al.* (1969): rats], the identification of foreign gammaglobulin proved to be analogous to our examinations.

A vast majority of our cases treated with ALG showed solely horse gammaglobulin at the glomerular BM. In cases 1, 5 and in the first biopsy of case 6, an identical pattern of deposits for the host's complement, in the sense of a complete heterologic phase of the Masugi nephritis, was found. Morphologically and clinically no criteria for a glomerulonephritis were revealed. Disregarding the effect of an additional immunosuppressive therapy, the reason for this presumably is that the ALG content of nephrotoxic antibodies is extremely low. To induce glomerulonephritis in Rhesus monkeys (MOPPERT *et al.*, 1970), we needed an amount of ALG as had been reached in our patients only after a therapy of several months' duration. On the other hand, it is known that a tenth of the amount of antibodies needed to induce nephritis in rats can be disclosed at the glomerula by immunohistology.

Case 11 and the third biopsy of case 10 immunohistologically showed the complete picture of an autologous phase of Masugi nephritis. In case 11, immunosuppressive therapy with azathioprine had been discontinued for reasons of intolerance 7 months before the first biopsy. The recipient's production of antibodies against the glomerularly fixed ALG did, even in these cases, not lead to morphologic signs of glomerulonephritis: in case 11, there had been an extremely severe TGP in the first biopsy. In case 10, the glomerula were almost unchanged as compared with the two earlier biopsies.

That case 10 produced antibodies against ALG at the time of the third biopsy could also be seen in the fact that the picture of an immunocomplex nephritis with granular deposits of horse gammaglobulin, host's complement and -IgM was additionally found at the BM by immunohistology. Clinically, a considerable proteinuria existed at that time which abated distinctly after discontinuation of ALG.

Glomerularly fixed ALG is obviously decomposed very slowly. Thus, we could identify by immunohistology horse gammaglobulin at the glomerular basement membranes even $4^1/_2$ (case 15) and 15 months resp. (case 5) after discontinuation of the ALG therapy.

The central question confronting us, is whether the described immunofluorescent findings in TGP are also the structural manifestation of glomerulonephritis. Apart from a relapse of the primary disease, a glomerulonephritis developed de novo — possibly as a result of the formation of transplant antibodies under ALG medication — would have to be taken into consideration.

Apart from observation 3, we could find no morphologically definite glomerulonephritic criteria. Particularly the light-optic preparations show no regular hypercellularity (on the contrary cf. GLASSOCK *et al.*, 1968). We missed dense synechias, which can prove glomerulonephritis if vascular diseases are excluded (cf. also IWASAKI *et al.*, 1967), in all cases but observation 3. Only in one observation (Fig. 11) we found a BM picture, which might be approximately equivalent to nephrotoxic Masugi nephritis. All other cases lacked such a change. In this connection we must emphasize again that the finely-granular, very loose subendothelial formations of pads, or rather thickenings of the internal lamina rara, are not equivalent to any picture of glomerulonephritis known by experiments. They are, however, at least very much alike glomerulo-nephrotic changes (hepatic, forms induced by radiation, leptospirosis ictero-hemorrhagica, see below). The observation of humps, which we could not find in our material, would prove acute diffuse glomerulonephritis of the immuno-complex type (serum sickness). However, it must be admitted, that humps disappear also in a trivial streptococcical glomerulonephritis after 6 weeks on the average. All our cases lack a severe proliferative change of the mesangium and endothelium. Besides, we did not find the tendency towards obliteration of glomerula as seen after a glomerulonephritic attack, but we observed vas-cularly-induced glomerular collapse with final hyaline glomerular scars. Hume et al. (1970) attach great importance to the electron-dense subendo-thelial deposits, which we did not find in all cases. We also missed the scars left by primary glomerulonephritis. On the other hand, electron-dense sub-endothelial deposits appear in other diseases of the kidney as well. In our opinion, the existence of glomerulonephritis cannot be diagnosed from these osmiophilic deposits, as similar deposits can also be found in hepatic glomerulo-nephrosis and X-ray glomerulopathy without presence of inflammatory changes.

Though we must admit that the differentiation of glomerulonephritis from TGP is not easy (cf. also Hume et al., 1970; Glassock et al., 1968; Porter et al., 1967; Dixon et al., 1969), we are thoroughly convinced that, with the exception of observation 3, there was no glomerulonephritis among the cases at issue.

The changes of the internal lamina rara, which show continuously in all our cases, cannot be taken as a manifestation of glomerulonephritis. The argument, it might be a modified form of glomerulonephritis under the in-fluence of immunosuppressives, is not valid. The publications on immuno-suppressive treatment in primary glomerulonephritis, known up to date, do not describe any analogous changes. Besides, the change of the lamina rara in observation 11 is very distinct, though immunosuppressives had been dis-continued 7 months before the first and 12 months before the second biopsy.

Most statements in literature (Hamburger et al., 1964; Hume et al., 1970: 12 out of 140, Rossmann et al., 1970: 2 out of 32, Busch et al., 1971a: 1 out of 24) coincide with our only case of secured glomerulonephritis out of 21 transplant cases. We cannot decide, whether this one case shows a relapse of glomerulonephritis, or whether a spontaneous glomerulonephritis developed on grounds of transplant antibodies (Hamburger and Dormont, 1968; Hume et al., 1965).

After not having accepted the glomerulonephritic nature of TGP, we would like to reject a connection between ALG-medication on the one hand and TGP on the other, as equivalent changes in moderate to severe (cases 7, 3, 12) or rather slight form (cases 4, 2, 10, 16) were also observed without the administration of ALG. It is true, immunohistological changes in the sense of the homologous phase of Masugi nephritis, less frequently of complex type nephritis, appeared; but they did not lead to the development of a morphologically conspicuous glomerulonephritis or glomerulopathy, or rather to clinically significant functional damages (cf. also FRIES *et al.*, 1970; TRAEGER *et al.*, 1969; TRAEGER and FRIES, 1969; HUME *et al.*, 1970; STARZL *et al.*, 1967a, b; on the contrary cf. GILLE *et al.* (1970) and BUSCH *et al.* (1971 b).

The favourable effect of ALG as to survival time and pathologic-anatomic changes (GUTTMANN *et al.*, 1969; DE VRIES *et al.*, 1968, a.o.), also proved in animal experiments, is therefore not restricted by secondary glomerular damages. One must not forget that the observation of 3 cases with diffuse glomerulonephritis in man after treatment with horse anticancerous serum (DELAPAVA *et al.*, 1962), which usually are used as chief witnesses against ALG, is a considerably different matter, as immunosuppressives were not used.

Although we reject the inflammatory (glomerulonephritic) nature of TGP, the question concerning its pathogenesis still remains. Consequently it has been considered whether the host's transplant antibodies are continuously removed by the functioning transplant and also deposited at the glomerular BM (WILLIAMS *et al.*, 1968 b). PORTER *et al.* (1967) take this possibility into account, too, however stating at the same time that deposits of this kind are also caused by carbon tetrachloride, synthetic polysaccharides and many other substances without the involvement of a conspicuous immunologic process (cf. also ANDRES *et al.*, 1970). This coincides with our IF-findings. Surveying a larger series of cases with varying primary diseases and differing therapies, like ours, there is, at least morphologically, no common denominator. An exception is the finely granular, loose thickening of the internal lamina rara.

A significant involvement of corticoide in the development of TGP can be excluded according to the examinations of HUME *et al.* (1970) and other authors. Some authors attribute the thickening of the subendothelial internal lamina rara to the deposit of fibrin (LINDQUIST *et al.*, 1970a, b), where by fragments of platelets are possibly of importance too (PORTER *et al.*, 1967). This is indicated by the fact that the equivalent transplant vasculopathy, in which severe endothelial damage can be ascertained in the medium and larger arteries regularly at the time of rejection, is said to be remediable by heparine treatment (CLYNE *et al.*, 1969). Moreover, a fibrinuria, abating in the course of time, has been ascertained in 54% of all transplants; between its severity and that of the nephropathy developing lateron, a satisfactory correlation is said to exist (ANTOINE *et al.*, 1969). We could also ascertain by electron microscopy subendothelially scattered fibrinous elements in more or less good condition (cf. BUSCH *et al.*, 1971 a). This identification was more frequently successful by immunohistochemistry. In one observation (11), we could identify light-optically coarse fibrinous beams in the extremely thickened internal lamina rara (Fig. 21). But on the whole, the significance of fibrin in the development of internal lamina rara changes seems to have been overvalued. We do not believe that the deposition of fibrin, in particular, is important, but we think, that plasma constituents, in a broad sense, are decisive for the change of the membrane. Manuel et al. (1967) believe the result of ischaemia being present. We object to this, because we could never observe analogous changes in central arterial contraction of the kidney.

Attention has repeatedly been called to the similarity of TGP to glomerulopathy in affections of the liver. In the latter, a thickening of the BM, or rather of the internal lamina rara, with subendothelial deposits of loose, finely granular material can be observed, which seems to change into osmiophilic deposits later on (Sakaguchi et al., 1964, 1965; Jones et al., 1961; Pierce and Nakane, 1969). As to cause, the hepatic genesis of TGP does not seem to come into question, for in our series there was only one severe disease of the liver (case 3) with dystrophy of short duration proving fatal. In this disease we have never observed changes of the kidney of such a kind. The severe hepatic glomerulopathy develops only in liver insufficiency of long duration. A low-grade hepatopathy existed in observation 16.

Especially striking is the similarity of TGP to radiation glomerulopathy, in which a new membrane between the finely granular masses and the endothelium may develop, such as described above (Madrazo et al., 1969, 1970; Rosen et al., 1968; Rosen and Cole, 1969). As to our material, we would object to X-ray damages explaining TGP in general. Cases without kidney radiation (3, 11, 15, 18) disclose TGP too (cf. also Hume et al., 1970). Under no circumstances is a dose of 300–1300 R sufficient to cause such severe glomerular changes by itself in the human (Zollinger, 1966). However, it cannot be excluded with certainty that radiation might have had an additional effect in the genesis of glomerulopathy, although in our opinion of minimum degree. It is interesting to note, that in X-ray glomerulopathy the endothelial damage and the secondary proliferation, which may lead to the occlusion of the loops, are in the foreground of the processes in the early phases (Mohr and Morgenroth, 1965). The endothelial damage is to be regarded as the cause of the BM alteration.

According to our recent observations, such a severe endothelial damage leads to a characteristic glomerulopathy in leptospirosis ictero-hemorrhagica (Zollinger et al., 1971); in this disease the endothelium of the intertubular and glomerular capillaries is the main aim of attack of the leptospirae. The result is a loosening and thickening of the internal lamina rara, which cannot be differentiated from TGP by electron microscopy. Even $4^1/_2$ months after the acute infection, ultrastructural membranous changes could be identified in this disease, although all clinical findings had become completely normal by that time.

In analogy to the two forms of disease mentioned, one finds in all cases of TGP degenerative and regenerative changes of the endothelial cells, probably lasting for years. These cells are mainly regarded as the target elements for the aggressive factors (cells or antibodies against HL-A antigen) in host reaction to transplants. It is imaginable that the endothelial lesion leads to secondary functional derangement of organisation in the wall of the loops, and tertiarily, to an increased permeability for serum elements, thus being the main factor in the pathogenesis of TGP. Whether the formation of thrombi, following the endothelial damage, is decisive for the development of TGP (BUSCH *et al.*, 1971a) seems questionable. On the other hand, the primary severe damage of the endothelium in early rejection cannot be doubted (HUME, 1969; HUME *et al.*, 1970; MERRILL, 1970; FELDMAN and SUN LEE, 1967; DEMPSTER *et al.*, 1964; WAKSMAN, 1963; KINCAID-SMITH, 1967; ROWLANDS *et al.*, 1967; PORTER *et al.*, 1965; ROSSMANN *et al.*, 1969; HUME, 1966; KIRKPATRICK and WILSON, 1964; RUSSELL *et al.*, 1969; LINDQUIST *et al.*, 1968a). This applies also to the intertubular vessels (FELDMAN and SUN LEE, 1967; ROWLANDS and BOSSEN, 1969; WILLIAMS *et al.*, 1964; PORTER *et al.*, 1964b). The interstitial edema is interpreted by most authors as secondary result of the endothelial damage and not as direct immunologic feature (LINDQUIST *et al.*, 1968a, WILLIAMS *et al.*, 1964b). This manifestation is valid for skin transplants as well. In his Fig. 9 GRUNDMANN (1970), e.g., shows rather similar acute lesions such as we found in acute renal rejection. Antigen antibody complexes can be identified in the walls of the blood-vessels (HOROWITZ *et al.*, 1963). Shortly before rejection, the humoral antibodies are much increased in the serum. Then they abate, a phenomenon, which has been explained by absorption in the blood vessels (ROWLANDS *et al.*, 1967). In our cases, we were able to prove endothelial lesions in the intertubular vessels analogous to the glomerular changes. Four times we found IgG and complement in the walls of the intertubular vessels.

The reasons given above make us assume, that low-grade episodes of rejection, which probably progress subclinically in most cases, occur in practically all kidney transplants over a period of years, and that they lead to endothelial damage with consecutive regeneration every time anew. BUSCH *et al.* (1971a) came to the same conclusion. In each process of such a damage, the serum elements, which are normally retained by the whole of the various loop elements, are able to permeate subendothelially and to reach the lamina densa. The reasons for their staying there are not yet known. If our theory of endothelial damage, due to an immunological mechanism followed by insudation and deposition with plasma elements, is correct, we should be able to find a correlation between histocompatibility and the severity of TGP. Indeed, if development of TGP is plotted against time (Fig. 1), each case seems to reach its specific maximum within the first 12 months and to remain constant thereafter. Since most of all rejection episodes occur during the first year, one is tempted to see a causal relationship between rejection or incompatibility and TGP. A closer look reveals a certain trend between incompatibility and TGP (Fig. 39, 40, 41), but the scatter is much too wide to allow any definite conclusion. Several factors, which possibly hide a true correlation, seem responsible for this scatter. First, incompatible kidneys were often only available for examination relatively early after transplantation when there was not enough time for TGP to develop. On the other hand, compatible kidneys could be followed with biopsies over much longer periods. Therefore, if time plays a role, this bias may account in part for the scatter in Fig. 39.

Second, patients with relatively incompatible grafts are treated with far more massive immunosuppression. Hence, the well-doing compatible grafts, where rejection remains subclinical, may be exposed to a weak immune attack over a long period without adequate immunosuppressive treatment. Such a long-lasting weak attack might lead to a similar endothelial damage as a much stronger, but heavily treated immune assault. Third, little is known about the mechanism for long-surviving allografts. If enhancing or blocking antibodies play a major role, the local deposition of such antibodies may prevent rejection without avoiding some morphological alterations. All these points explain the different opinions of several authors about this object. McPhaul et al. (1970) found a complete lack of correlation between histocompatibility and TGP, while other authors affirm certain connections (Peterson et al., 1966; Lindquist et al., 1970b; Fries et al., 1970; Porter et al., 1967; Hume et al., 1970; Harlan et al., 1967; Busch et al., 1968; Weymouth et al., 1970; Busch et al. 1971a).

The lacking correlation between the severity of TGP and the degree of proteinuria is especially striking. Sampling errors introduced with needle biopsy cannot exclusively account for these findings. Two specimens were taken at least with each biopsy. In cases where large specimens could be obtained in the same patient, either by open surgical biopsy or at the time of kidney removal, the findings did not differ substantially from the former examinations with needle biopsy specimens. Minimum to moderate proteinuria despite severe glomerular changes seem to be a characteristic feature of TGP. A nephrotic syndrome, which were often suspected when looking at the biopsy, did never occur. It must be presumed that the compact deposits in the internal endothelial rara of the BM are not always followed by a corresponding change of the physical property of the membrane.

The extreme difficulty to explain the different maximum degrees of TGP in the individual cases can only be overcome by making allowance for the second factor, namely therapy. In other words: Not the histo-incompatibility as such, but the resultant from the damaging factor (damage by incompatibility) and the reciprocal factor restricting the damage (effectivity of immunosuppression) is thought to be decisive for the development of the endothelial damage and, consequently, of TGP. If the damage-restricting factor of therapy is left out such as we observed in one case outside this series, the maximum degree of TGP develops as soon as 6 weeks after transplantation.

D. Summary

The morphogenesis of transplant-glomerulopathy (TGP) was examined by light, electron and immunofluorescence-microscopy in 30 biopsies and 7 grafted kidneys retrieved through operation or autopsy from a total of 20 cadaver kidney transplants. The results were compared with those of the pertinent literature.

The principal change in the case of TGP consists in an electron-loose subendothelial thickening of the internal lamina rara of the basement membrane (BM). The thickening of the whole BM can be more than 50 times its normal size. In such areas, cell organelles or whole cytoplasm processes are often embedded. Individual erythrocytes and/or fibrin threads resp. fragments are not found as often. In severe degrees of TGP lamina densa-like material will be found partly subendothelially in form of a newly developed lamina densa, partly as meshwork.

In 10 cases, subendothelial and/or mesangial osmiophilic deposits could be identified. They do not correlate with the primary kidney disease. Two biopsies of one case showed subepithelial osmiophilic deposits, which contain spherical inclusions of about 780 Å. In accordance with data of pertinent literature, they are interpreted as viruses.

The most important change of the cells pertains to the endothelium of the glomerular capillary loops and the intertubulary capillaries. In addition to proliferation, leading to almost total obliteration of the capillary lumen through endothelial cell processes, degenerative lesions were found.

The latter are especially prominent in the course of acute rejection phases. In a few cases, glomerular endothelial foam cells are being formed, such as are known in transplant vasculopathy.

The mesangial cells are only slightly multiplied. However, the mesangial matrix is increased (so-called BM-like substance). The processes of the visceral epithelium are often seen in increased numbers and edematously puffed. Fusion of foot processes is often found, but it changes in intensity from loop to loop. Substantial changes of the capsule are missing.

As the curves of the course show, the individually quite variable maximum degree of TGP is reached in about 5–12 months. It does not change considerably lateron. A relation between ALG-therapy and TGP does not seem to be present.

The immunohistological examination of the glomerula gave two results independent of each other:

1. More than 50% of the biopsies show granular to short-linear immunoglobular deposits (mainly IgM), mostly combined with C'3. Judging by the literature, it appears probable that these are soluble deposits of immunocomplexes whose pathogenesis however is not clear and probably not uniform. A definitive correlation between the immunohistological changes and the intensity of the glomerulopathy, noticeable by light- and electron-microscopy, does not exist in our observations.

2. The cases treated with ALG (intravenously with one exception) show a linear lining of the glomerular basement membrane with horse-gamma-globulins.

On the basis of our own investigations it can be proven that the above-mentioned findings result from contamination of the used ALG with an antibody fraction against basement membrane. In two patients, immunohisto-logical tests proved the existence of deposits and production of humoral antibodies against the given ALG. In spite of this, the ALG-therapy did not in any of our cases lead to a clearly recognizeable glomerulonephritis or to an intensification of the glomerulopathy.

A correlation between the severity of TGP and proteinuria cannot be proven. Remarkable in the first place is the very light proteinuria in spite of grave glomerular changes. Although the number of rejections, HL-A-compatibility and clinical compatibility-classification show a certain trend of conformity with the TGP degree, the deviations are too big to form an un-ambiguous opinion. On the other hand, it seems possible, that an existing causal relation between incompatibility and TGP is only veiled. Only in one case, a subacute extracapillary glomerulonephritis could be diagnosed. We are of the opinion, that the TGP does not correspond to the light- and ultrastruc-tural image of a glomerulonephritis. Comparisons with qualitatively similar glomerulopathies in leptospirosis ictero-hemorrhagica, chronical hepatic diseases and after exposure to ionizing radiation show, that an inflammatory lesion of the glomerular loops can be excluded.

It is assumed, that clinically known or occult episodes of rejection lead to relatively often repeated damage of the endothelium with following regeneration. By this, the functional qualities of the glomerular and intertubular capillary walls are injured, and plasmatic insudate is deposited in the area of the internal lamina rara. This results in the described glomerular alteration. The reason, why this material, unidentifyable in particular, cannot be eliminated furthermore, is not clear. According to this hypothesis, the TGP is the resultant of the histoincompatibility on one hand and the success of the immune suppression on the other. As these two factors vary very much, it is not surprising, that a distinct relation between the degree of histoincompatibility and the TGP was not found.

References

Andres, G. A., Accinni, L., Hsu, K. C., Penn, I., Porter, K. A., Rendall, I. M., Seegal, B. C., Starzl, T. E.: Human renal transplants, III. Immunopathologic studies. Lab. Invest., **22**, 588–604 (1970).

Antoine, B., Neveu, T., Ward, T.: Fibrinuria in human renal transplants. Rev. franç. Étud. clin. biol. 14/8, 744–753 (1969).

Arakawa, M., Kimmelstiel, P.: Circumferential mesangial interposition. Lab. Invest. **21**, 276–248 (1969).

Bariéty, J., Druet, Ph., Samarcq, P., Lagrue, G.: Histogenèse des glomérulopathies «extra-membraneuses». J. Urol. Néphrol., **75**, 627–636 (1969).

Bariéty, J., Samarcq, P., Lagrue, L., Fritel, D., Milliez, P.: Evolution ultrastructurale favorable de deux cas de glomérulopathies primitives à dépòts extra-membraneux diffus. Presse méd. **76**, 2179–2182 (1968).

Busch, G. J., Braun, W. J., Glassock, R. J., Dammin, G. J.: Immunofluorescent patterns in human renal allografts. Lab. Invest. 18, 321 (1968).

Busch, G. J., Galvanek, E. G., Reynolds, E. S.: Human renal allografts. Analysis of lesions in long term survivors. Human pathology 2, 253–298 (1971a).

Busch, G. J., Kobayashi, K., Birtch, A. G., Galvanek, E. G., Lukl, P., Jr., Carpenter, Ch. B.: Human renal allografts: Glomerular deposition of horse immunoglobulin G and nephritis following administration of antilymphocyte globuline. Human pathology 2, 299–308 (1971b).

CHURG, J., GRISHHAM, E.: Subacute glomerulonephritis. Amer. J. Path. **35**, 25–32 (1959).

CLYNE, D. H., KINCAID-SMITH, P., MARSHALL, V. C., MORRIS, P. J.: Anticoagulants in the treatment of patients with renal allografts; modification of the vascular lesions of rejections. Abstracts IVth Internat. Congress Nephrology, p. 328, Stockholm 1969.

COHEN, B. J., DE VRIES, M. J., VAN NOORD, M. J., LUBBE, F. H.: Stain-specific renal toxicity of heterologous antilymphocyte γ-globulin in mice. Transplant. **10**, 1–19 (1970).

CROSNIER, J.: Les complications immunologiques rénales de la transplantation du rein. J. Urol. Néphrol. **75**, 12, 237–240 (1969).

DEMPSTER, W. J., HARRISON, C. V., SHACKMAN, R.: Rejection processes in human homotransplanted kidneys. Brit. med. J., 1964, II, 969–976.

DIXON, F. J., McPHAUL, J. J., JR., LERNER, R. A.: Recurrence of glomerulonephritis in the transplanted kidney. Arch. intern. Med. **123**, 554–563 (1969).

EHRENREICH, T., CHURG, J.: Pathology of membranous nephropathy. In S. C. Sommers: Pathology annual, **3**, pg. 145–186. New York: Appleton-Century-Crafts, 1968.

FAITH, G. C., TRUMP, B. F.: The glomerular capillary wall in human kidney disease: acute glomerulonephritis, systemic lupus erythematodes, and preeclampsia-eclampsia. Lab. Invest. **15**, 1682–1719 (1966).

FELDMANN, J. D., SUN LEE: Renal homotransplantation in rats. I. Allogeneic recipients. J. exp. Med. **120**, 783–794 (1967).

FISH, A. J., HERDMANN, R. C., KELLY, W. D., GOOD, R. A.: Long term pathological alteration in well-functioning human renal homotransplants. Abstracts 3rd Intern. Congress Nephrology, Washington (1966), Transplantation **5**, 1334–1343 (1967).

FRIES, D., BLANC-BRUNAT, N., TRAEGER, J.: Pathology of renal allografts in patients receiving long-term antilymphocyte globuline therapy. Transpl. (Baltimore) **10**, 20–32 (1970).

GILLE, J., ZOBL, H., KRAUSE, P. H., GEORGII, A.: Immun-histologische Befunde an menschlichen Transplantatnieren. Verh. dtsch. Ges. Path. **54**, 653 (1970).

GLASSOCK, R. J., FELDMANN, D., REYNOLDS, E. S., DAMMIN, G. J., MERRILL, J. P.: Human renal isografts: a clinical and pathologic analysis. Medicine (Baltimore) **47**, 411–454 (1968).

GRUNDMANN, E.: Die Immunopathlogie der experimentellen Allo- und Xenotransplantation. Verh. dtsch. Ges. Path. **54**, 65–94 (1970).

GUTTMANN, R. D., LINDQUIST, R. R., OCKNER, S. S.: Renal transplantation in the inbred rat. XII. A mechanism of long-term survival of allografts after antithymocyte immunoglobulin treatment. Transpl. (Baltimore) **8**, 837–845 (1969).

HAMBURGER, J., CROSNIER, J., DORMONT, J.: Observations in patients with well-tolerated homotransplanted kidney: possibility of secondary disease. Ann. N.Y. Acad. Sci. **120**, 558–577 (1964).

HAMBURGER, J., CROSNIER, J., DORMONT, J.: La transplantation rénale. Proc. 3rd int. Cong. Nephrol. Washington 1966, vol. 3, 365–382 Basel-New York Karger, 1967.

HAMBURGER, J., DORMONT, J.: Functional and morphological alterations in long-term kidney transplants. In; F. T. RAPAPORT AND J. DAUSSET: Human transplantation, New York: Grune and Strattn, 1968, p. 201.

HAMBURGER, J., RICHET, G., CROSNIER, J., FUNK-BRENTANO, J. L., ANTOINE, B., DUCROT, H., MERRY, J. P., MONTERA, H. DE: Nephrology.vol. **2**, pg. 1296ff. Saunders, Philadelphia, London, Toronto :1968.

HARLAN, W. R., JR., HOLDEN, K. R., WILLIAMS, G. M., HUME, D. M.: Proteinuria and nephrotic syndrome associated with chronic rejection of kidney transplants. New Engl. J. Med. **277**, 769–772 (1967).

HOROWITZ, R. E., BURROWS, L., PARONETTO, F., WILDSTEIN, W.: Immunocytochemical observations on canine kidney homografts. Fed. Proc. **22**, 274 (1963).

HUME, D. M.: Renal homotransplantation in man: studies in 63 cases. In: F. K. MOSTOFI and D. E. SMITH: The kidney. Baltimore: Williams and Wilkins, 1966.

HUME, D. M.: Prospects of kidney transplantations. In: N. A. MITCHISON, J. M. GREEP and J. C. HALTINGA-VERSCHURE: Organ-transplantation. p. 311–326. Excerpta Med. Found., Amsterdam: 1969,

HUME, D. M., STERLING, W. A., WEYMOUTH, R. J., SIEBEL, H. R., MADGE, G. E., LEE, H. M.: Glomerulonephritis in human renal homotransplants. Transpl. Proceed. **2**, 361–412 (1970).

Irino, T., Hamamoto, Y.: Three types of productive glomerulitis. Jap. J. Nephrol. 8, 165–179 (1966).

Iwasaki, Y., Porter, K. A., Amend, J. R., Marchioro, T. L., Zuhle, V., Starzl, T. E.: The preparation and testing of horse anti-dog and anti-human antilymphoid plasma or serum and its protein fraction. Surg. Gynec. Obstet. 124, 1–12 (1967).

Jeannet, M., Weck, A. de, Grob, P., Thiel, G.: A cooperative kidney typing and exchange programm. Helvet. med. Acta 35, 239–247 (1967/70).

Jeannet, M., Weck, A. de, Grob, P., Horrisberger, B., Largiadèr, F., Thiel, G.: HL-A typing and cadavre-kidney transplants. Transpl. Proceed. 3, 1015–1018 (1971).

Jones, W. A., Govinda Rao, D. R., Braunstein, H.: The renal glomerulus in cirrhoses of the liver. Amer. J. Path. 39, 393–408 (1961).

Kano, K., Milgrom, F.: Relation of anti-γ-globulin antibodies to transplantation antibodies in huma renal allograft recipients. Transpl. 7, 281–289 (1969).

Kincaid-Smith, P.: Histological diagnosis of rejection of renal homografts in man. Lancet 1967 II, 849–852.

Kirkpatrick, Ch. H., Wilson, W. E.: Immunologic studies of Baboon-to-man renal heterotransplantation. In: T. E. Starzl: Experience in renal transplantation, pc. 284 Philadelphia and London: Saunders, 1964.

Krieg, A. F., Bolande, R. P., Holden, W. D., Hubay, C. H., Persky, L.: Membranous glomerulonephritis occuring in a human renal homotransplant. Amer. J. clin. Path. 34, 155–162 (1960).

Lindquist, R. R., Guttmann, R. D., Carpenter, C. B., Merrill, J. P.: Nephritis induced by antilymphocyte serum. Transpl. 8, 545–557 (1969a).

Lindquist, R. R., Guttmann, R. D., Mahabir, R. N.: Fibrin deposition as a pathogenetic mechanism producing glomerulopathy in long surviving renal allografts. Transpl. 9, 65–68 (1970).

Lindquist, R. R., Guttmann, R. D., Merrill, J. P.: Renal transplantation in the inbred rat. Amer. J. Path. 52, 531–545 (1868b).

Lindquist, R. R., Guttmann, R. D., Merrill, J. P.: Mononuclear (lymphoid) cells in rejecting renal allografts. Amer. J. Path. 55, 58a (1969b).

Lindquist, R. R., Guttmann, R. D., Merrill, J. P.: Renal transplantation in the inbred rat. VII. Ultrastructure of the glomerulus during acute renal allograft rejection. Transpl. 11, 1–9 (1971).

Lindquist, R. R., Guttmann, R. D., Merrill, J. P., Dammin, G. J.: Human renal allografts. Interpretation of morphologic and immunohistochemical observations. Amer. J. Path. 58, 851–867 (1968a).

Madrazo, A., Suzuki, Y., Churg, J.: Radiation nephritis. Acute changes following high dosis of radiation. Amer. J. Med. 54, 507–527 (1969).

Madrazo, A., Suzuki, Y., Churg, J.: Radiation nephritis. II. chronic changes after high doses of radiation. Amer. J. Path. 61, 39–56 (1970).

Manuel, Y., Poli, S., Bernhardt, J. P., Revillard, J. P., Claudy, D., Traeger, J.: Proteinuria in human renal allografts. Helv. med. Acta 35, 3–19 (1969).

McManus, J. F., Lupton, Ch. H.: Patterns of glomerular reaction. In: F. K. Mostofi and D. E. Smith: The kidney, p. 95–113. Baltimore: Williams and Wilkins, 1966.

McPhaul, J. J., Jr., Dixon, F. J., Brettschneider, L., Starzl, T. E.: Immunofluorescent examinations of biopsies from long-term renal allografts. New. Engl. J. Med. 282, 412–415 (1970).

Merrill, J. P.: Recent advances in nephrology-immunology. Proc. 4th Inter. Congr. of Nephrol. Stockholm, 1969, vol. 3, p. 8–22, Basel, München, New York: Karger 1970.

Milgrom, F., Klassen, J., Fuji, H.: Immunologic injury of renal homografts. J. exp. Med. 134, 1933–2079 (1971).

Mohr, H. J., Morgenroth, K.: Nierengewebsveränderungen nach gezielter hochdosierter Röntgenbestrahlung. Verh. dtsch. Ges. Path. 49, 206–211 (1965).

Moppert, J., Bühler, F., Thiel, G., Vischer, T., Zollinger, H. U.: Glomeruläre Fixation einer ALG-Komponente in menschlichen Nierentransplantaten. Verh. dtsch. Ges. Path. 54, 159–162 (1970).

Orr, W. McN., Birtch, A. G., Diethelm, A. G., Dubernard, J. M., Duguella, J., Glassock, R. G.: A study of the potential nephrotoxicity of heterologous antilymphocyte serum. Clin. exper. Immunol. 6, 305–311 (1970).

PAVA, S. DE LA, NIGOGOSYAN, G., PICKREN, J. W.: Fatal glomerulonephritis after receiving horse anti-human-cancer serum. Arch. intern. Med. **109**, 391–398 (1962).

PETERSON, E. W., McPHAUL, J. J., McINTOSH, D. A.: Serial histological alteration in human renal homotransplant. Amer. J. clin. Path. **45**, 521–532 (1966).

PIERCE, G. B., NAKANE, P. K.: Basement membranes. Synthesis and deposition in response to cellular injury. Lab. Invest. **21**, 27–41 (1969).

PORTER, K. A., ANDRES, G. A., CALDER, M. W., DOSSETOR, J. B., HSU, K. C., RENDALL, J. M., SEEGAL, B. C., STARZL, T. E.: Human renal transplants. II. Immunofluorescent and immunoferritin studies. Lab. Invest. **18**, 159–171 (1968).

PORTER, K. A., CALNE, R. Y., ZUKOSKI, C. F.: Vascular and other changes in 200 canine renal homotransplants treated with immunosuppressive drugs. Lab. Invest. **13**, 809–824 (1964a).

PORTER, K. A., DOSSETOR, J. B., MARCHIORO, T. L., PEART, W. S., RENDALL, J. M., STARZL, T. E., TERASAKI, P. I.: Human renal transplants. I. Glomerular changes. Lab. Invest. **16**, 153–181 (1967).

PORTER, K. A., JOSEPH, J. H., RENDALL, J. M., STOLINSKI, C., HOEHN, R. J., CALNE, R. Y.: The role of lymphocytes in the rejection of canine renal homotransplants. Lab. Invest. **13**, 1080–1098 (1964b).

PORTER, K. A., MARCHIORO, T. L., STARZL, T. E.: Pathological changes in 37 human renal homotransplants treated with immunosuppressive drugs. Brit. J. Urol. **37**, 250–273 (1965).

PORTER, K. A., THOMSOM, W. B., OWEN, K., KENYON, J. R., MOWBRAY, J. F., PEART, S. W.: Obliterative vascular changes in four human kidney homotransplants. Brit. med. J. (1963) **II**, 639–645.

RAPAPORT, F. T., DAUSSET, J.: Ranks of donor-recipient histocompatibility for human transplantation. Science **167**, 1260–1261 (1970).

ROSEN, V. J., COLE, L. C.: Radiation induced renal lesions in the rhodent. In E. BAJUSZ and G. JASMIN, Meth. Achiev. exper. Path. **4**, 214–236. 1969.

ROSEN, V. J., COLE, L. J., WACHTEL, L. W., DOGGETT, R. S.: Ultrastructural studies of X-ray induced glomerular disease in rats subjected to uninephrectomy and food restriction. Lab. Invest. **18**, 260–268 (1968).

ROSENAU, W., LEE, J. C., NAJARIAN, J. S.: A light, fluorescence and electron microscopic study of functionning human renal transplants. Surg. Gynec. Obstet. **128**, 62–76 (1969).

ROSSMANN, P., JIRKA, J., BROD, J., MALEK, P.: Histologie und Feinstruktur der Biopsien allotransplantierter Nieren. Beitr. path. Anat. **138**, 377–404 (1969).

ROSSMANN, P., JIRKA, J., RENELTOVA, I., MALEK, P., HEJNAL, J.: Histology and ultrastructure of recurrent glomerulonephritis in human allotransplanted kidneys. Beitr. path. Anat. **141**, 213–226 (1970).

ROUILLER, CH.: General anatomy and histology of the kidney. In: CH. ROUILLER and A. F. MÜLLER, The kidney vol. 1, p. 61–156. New York: Academic Press, 1969.

ROWLANDS, D. T., BOSSEN, E. H.: Immunological mechanisms of allograft rejection. Arch. Int. Med. **113**, 491–500 (1969).

ROWLANDS, D. T., BURKHOLDER, P. M., BOSSEN, E. H., LIN HSHU-HSLING: Renal allografts in HL-A matched recipients. Amer. J. Path. **61**, 177–210 (1970).

ROWLANDS, D. T., KIRKPATRICK, CH. H., VALTER, A. F., WILSON, W. E.: Immunologic studies in human organ transplantation. IV. Serologic and pathologic studies following heterotransplantation of the kidney. Amer. J. Path. **50**, 605–622 (1967).

RUSSELL, P. S.: Kidney transplantation. Amer. J. Med. **44**, 776–785 (1968).

RUSSELL, P. S., AUSTIN, K. F., FLAX, M. H., WINN, A. J.: Clinical immunopathology of renal transplantation. In: P. A. MIESCHER, H. J. MÜLLER-EBERHARD Textbook of immunopathology II, p. 752–767, New York: Grune and Stratton, 1969.

SAKAGUCHI, H., DACHS, S., MAUTNER, W., GRISHMAN, E., CHURG, J.: Renal glomerular lesions after administration for carbon tetrachloride and athionine. Lab. Invest. **13**, 1418–1426 (1964).

SAKAGUCHI, H., DACHS, S., PARONETTO, F., SALOMON, M., CHURG, J.: Hepatic glomerulosclerosis: An electron microscopic study of renal biopsies in liver disease. Lab. Invest. **14**, 533–545 (1965).

Simon, G. T., Chatelanat, F.: Ultrastructure of the normal and pathological glomerulus. In: Ch. Rouiller, A. F. Müller: The kidney vol. I, p. 261–349. Academic Press, NewYork 1969.

Starzl, T. E., Marchioro, T. L., Porter, K. A., Iwasaki, Y., Cerilli, G. J.: The use of heterologous agents in canine liver homotransplantation and in human renal transplantation. Surg. Gynec. Obstetr. **124**, 301–324 (1967a).

Starzl, T. E., Porter, K. A, Iwasaki, Y., Marchioro, T. L., Kashiwagi, N.: The use of heterologous antilymphocyte globulin in human renal homotransplantation. In: G. E. Wolstenholme and M. O'Connor, Antilymphocytic serum. Ciba Foundation Study Group Nr 29 Boston Little, Brown & Co., 1967b.

Stocker, J. W., McKenzie, I. F. C., Morris, P. J.: IgM activity in human lymphotoxic antisera after renal transplantation. Nature (Lond.) **222**, 483–484 (1969).

Strunk, S. W., Hammond, W. S., Benditt, E. P.: The resolution of acute glomerulonephritis. An electron microscopic study of four sequental biopsies. Lab. Invest. **13**, 401–429 (1964).

Thiel, G.: Problèmes cliniques de l'immunosuppression chez les patients subissant une transplantation rénale. Méd. et Hyg. **27**, 1487–1491 (1969).

Thiel, G., Moppert, J., Mahlich, J., Bühler, F., Vischer, T., Enderlin, F., Weber, H., Zollinger, H. U.: Glomerular damage after intravenous administration of antilymphocyte globulin (ALG) in man and rhesus monkeys. Transplant. Proceed. **3**, 741—744 (1971).

Traeger, J., Fries, D., Revillard, J. P., Brochnier, J., Brunat-Blanc, M.: Antilymphocytic globulins in kidney transplantation. Effects on glomerular disease. Transpl. Proceed. **1**, 1006–1012 (1969).

Traeger, J., Fries, F.: Expérience clinique avec le sérum antilymphocytaire. J. Urol. Néphrol. **75**, 200–210 (1969).

Vries, M. J. de, Tinbergen, W. J., Westbroek, D. L.: The effect of various immunosuppressive agents on the histology of the homograft reaction. VIIth Int. Congr. Int. Acad. Pathol., Milan 1968, p. 72–73.

Waksman, B. H.: The pattern of rejection in rat skin homografts, and its relationship to the vascular network. Lab. Invest. **12**, 46–57 (1963).

Weymouth, R. J., Seibel, H. R., Lee, H. M., Hume, D. M., Williams, G. M.: The glomerulus in man one hour after transplantation: an electron microscopic study. Amer. J. Path. **58**, 85–104 (1970).

Williams, G. M., Hume, D. M., Hudson, P., Jr., Morris, P. J., Kano, K., Milgrom, F.: New Engl. J. Med. **279**, 611–616 (1968a).

Williams, G. M., Hume, D. M., Kano, K., Milgrom, F.: Transplantation antibodies in human recipients of renal homografts. J. Amer. med. Assoc. **204**, 119–122 (1968b).

Williams, P. L., Williams, M. A., Kountz, S. L., Dempster, W. J.: Ultrastructural and haemodynamic studies in canine renal transplants. J. Anat. (Lond.) **98**, 545–569 (1964).

Zollinger, H. U.: Niere und ableitende Harnwege. In: W. Doerr und E. Uehlinger: Spezielle pathologische Anatomie. Bd. 3, Berlin, Heidelberg, New York: Springer; 1966.

Zollinger, H. U., Colombi, A., Schiltknecht, J.: New clinical and ultrastructural aspects in leptospirosis icterohaemorrhagica (Weil's disease). Virchow Archiv **354**, 336–348 (1971).

Zollinger, H. U., Rohr, H. P.: Struktur und Bedeutung der renalen Schaumzellen. Virchows Arch. Abt. A. **348**, 205–219 (1969).

Department of Pathology, Columbia University, College of Physicians and Surgeons, and the Francis Delafield Hospital New York, New York 10032

Some Aspects of Sarcoidosis

HENRY A. AZAR, EDWARD A. MOSCOVIC, SOLANGE G. ABUNASSAR, and J. STEVEN McDOUGAL

With 14 Figures

Contents

I. Introduction: Definition and Scope

Sarcoidosis continues to present one of the most controversial and challenging problems of human pathology. In spite of recent intensive epidemiological, clinical, immunological and ultrastructural studies, the nature of sarcoidosis appears to be presently as elusive as when described by HUTCHINSON, BOECK, BESNIER and SCHAUMANN. The more recent historical sketches of JAMES (1968) and BUCKLEY (1970) bring into perspective the difficulties encountered over the past hundred years in defining this condition of unknown etiology and pathogenesis.

The following review is not meant to be an authoritative and complete account of developments in the field of sarcoidosis. Such updated and comprehensive reviews are found in the Proceedings of International Conferences on Sarcoidosis, particularly the 3rd and 4th Conferences, edited respectively by Löfgren (1964), and by Turiaf and Chabot (1967). The reviews of Siltzbach (1968, 1969) are also an excellent source of information. An exhaustive literature search on sarcoidosis from mid-1963 to mid-1966 has been compiled by the National Library of Medicine at Bethesda.

This paper will deal primarily with morphologic aspects of sarcoidosis but will also touch on other aspects of this condition which are relevant to the pathogenesis and possible nature of the sarcoid lesion. A definition of sarcoidosis at this time is impossible to achieve because of fundamental gaps in our knowledge. At most, we can speak here of an anatomic and clinical syndrome which, for our purposes, may be defined as a non-necrotizing, non-caseating, epithelioid, granulomatous reaction in which no etiologic agent can be identified by our present means. To this definition, one may add that the lesions are often seen in nodes of the neck, and mediastinum but may involve the lungs, the skin, the uveal tract or parotid glands. Sarcoid lesions have been described in almost all parts of the body, with the possible exception of the adrenal gland, and may include, according to some authors (Mitchell et al., 1970), Crohn's disease. Sarcoid-like reactions have been described in relation to a variety of malignant neoplasms, particularly Hodgkin's disease (Brinker, 1970). One must also add that patients with widespread and active sarcoid lesions often exhibit a state of relative anergy or diminished delayed hypersensitivity reactions to sensitizing agents such as tuberculin, and react positively to the subcutaneous injection of the Kveim antigen (Siltzbach, 1967).

II. Morphologic Basis of Sarcoidosis
A. The Sarcoid Granuloma

Morphologically, sarcoidosis is characterized by a granulomatous reaction ranging in extent from a localized lesion to disseminated forms, all manifested by discrete or confluent epithelioid granulomas which bear a striking resemblance to classical tuberculous granulomas. Unlike the latter, there is, as a rule, minimal or no necrosis, and, by definition, no caseation necrosis. Depending on the age of the lesion, the sarcoid reaction may be totally epithelioid with no, or few, multinucleated giant cells of the Langhans type, or may exhibit varying degrees of collagenization or hyalinosis with obliteration of the underlying epithelioid appearance.

The epithelioid cells may be surrounded by or intermingle with lymphocytes, plasma cells, fibroblasts and, less commonly, histiocytes or macrophages. In lymph nodes and, more particularly, in the spleen, the relationship of the sarcoidal lesion to small blood vessels, including arterioles, is often quite evident. Almost all tissues in the body may be affected, but involvement of the central nervous system is uncommon and that of the adrenal glands seem to have been left out in accounts of histologic studies of sarcoidosis. This may, of course, bear some biological significance since the blood-brain barrier may be effective in blocking the entrance of cells or agents involved in sarcoid granulomas, whereas the adrenal glands, because of their glucosteroid content, may hinder the establishment of noninfectious granulomas.

B. The Epithelioid Cell; Derivation

The term epithelioid (epithelial-like) is derived from the superficial resemblance of the major cell population of sarcoid granulomas to closely-packed parenchymal cells. The term, "epithelioid", in spite of its awkwardness, is a convenient one; its use led us to avoid for decades a meaningful confrontation with the problem of derivation of these cells. Epithelioid cells do not behave like macrophages since they seldom display any significant phagocytic ability. In fields of anthracosis or of old hemorrhage, they seldom pick up any carbon or hemosiderin particles. In our experience with caseating tuberculous granulomas, mycobacteria as demonstrated by fluorescent staining (WILNER et al., 1969) were rarely seen in significant numbers except in caseous areas and in zones bordering areas of caseation. "Hard" epithelioid tubercles of patients known to have tuberculosis rarely contain mycobacteria. The lack of avid phagocytosis on the part of epithelioid cells does not preclude, however, the possibility that they are impotent macrophages.

Epithelioid cells are closely packed, and have ill-defined boundaries. Their cytoplasm is usually light staining or may exhibit various shades of eosinophilia or even slight basophilia. The nuclei are generally ovoid or indented, and vesicular. Their appearance is closer to that of macrophages and fibroblasts than to that of small lymphocytes and plasma cells. The multinucleated giant cells formed in epithelioid granulomas share the cytoplasmic and nuclear properties of epithelioid cells.

The ultrastructure of the epithelioid cells of sarcoidosis has been intensively studied, among others, by GUSEK (1964, 1966), WANSTRUP and CHRISTENSEN (1966), WANSTRUP (1968), HIRSCH et al. (1967) and KALIFAT et al. (1967). Under the electron microscope, the epithelioid cells manifest an unsuspected degree of variation in their cellular detail. Some are rich in multiple vesicles and pinocytic vacuoles, as well as presence of membrane-bound dense granules of varying size. Others have a markedly developed endoplasmic reticulum comparable to that of plasma cells or fibroblasts. Mitochondria are usually present in large numbers and show varying degrees of degenerative changes such as ballooning, and loss of cristae. Dense, intramitochondrial granules are frequently seen (LUNARDELLI, 1968). It is not clear whether epithelioid cells belong to several types, types resembling reticular cells or histiocytes, stimulated lymphocytes or fibroblasts, or whether various components of the cytoplasm of an epithelioid cells contain features of the above cited cell lines. The cytoplasmic borders of epithelioid cells are frequently villous in character and neighboring cells show an intricate intertwining of their peripheral cell processes. Representative fine structural features of epithelioid are shown in Fig. 1.

4*

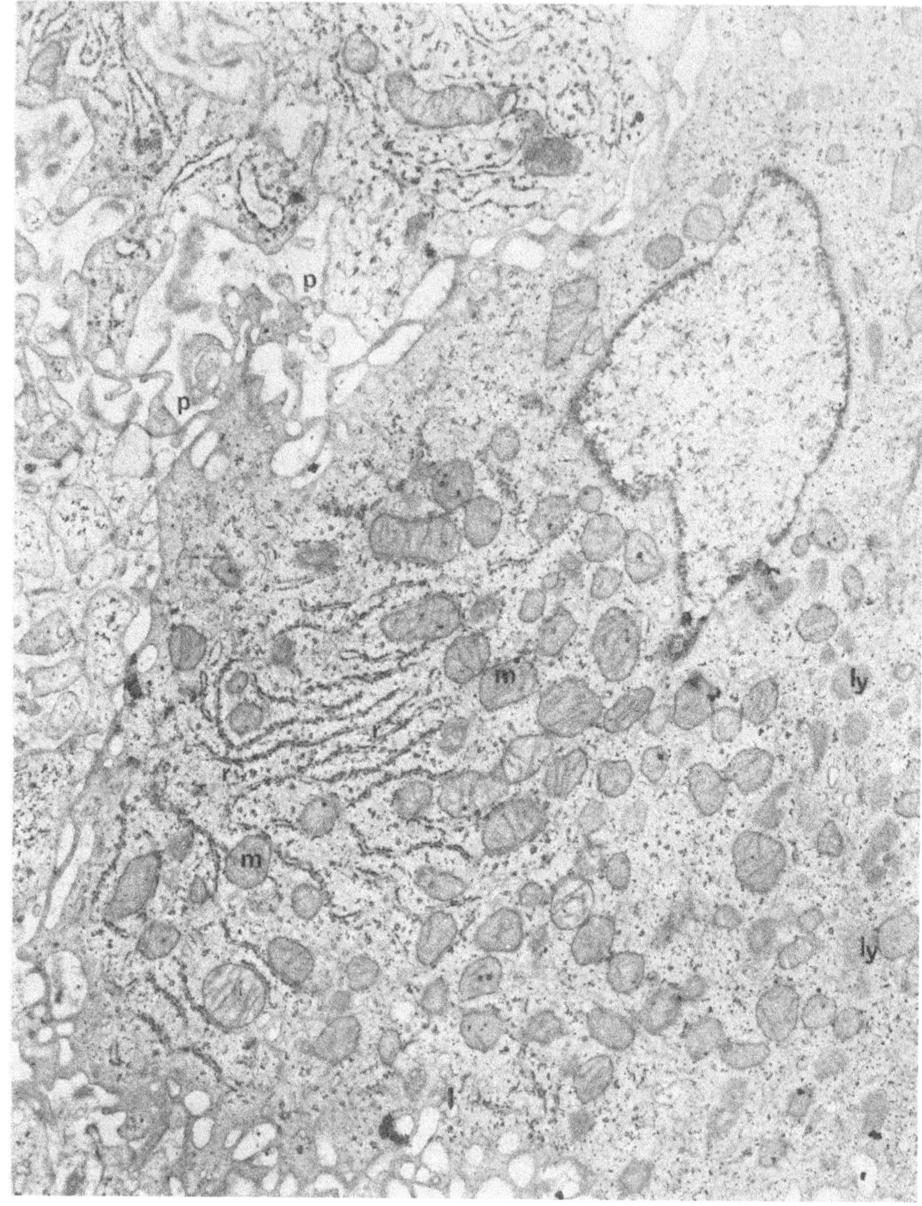

Fig. 1. Portion of epithelioid cell. Note abundance of mitochondria (*m*), membrane-bound lysozomal granules (*ly*), rough endoplasmic reticulum (*r*) and peripheral cell processes (*p*). × 28800. This and subsequent electron microscope preparations were stained with uranyl acetate and lead citrate

The formation of multinucleated giant cells appears to be the result of partial loss of limiting cell membranes. Segments of parallel cell membranes often persist within the cytoplasm of multinucleated giant cells suggesting that the giant cells are the result of syncytial fusion of neighboring epithelioid cells (Azar and Lunardelli, 1969) (Fig. 2, 3).

As to the derivation of epithelioid cells, it is tempting to consider that each epithelioid granuloma is derived from a progenitor cell, or small group of cells, blood-derived, which have proliferated in response to a locally-trapped, triggering agent. Of course, today, it is not inconceivable to think of some lymphocytes as pluri-potential lymphoreticular cells capable of both *in vivo* and *in vitro* transformation into larger blastoid forms. It has been well-documented that peripheral lymphocytes incubated with phytohemagglutinin will

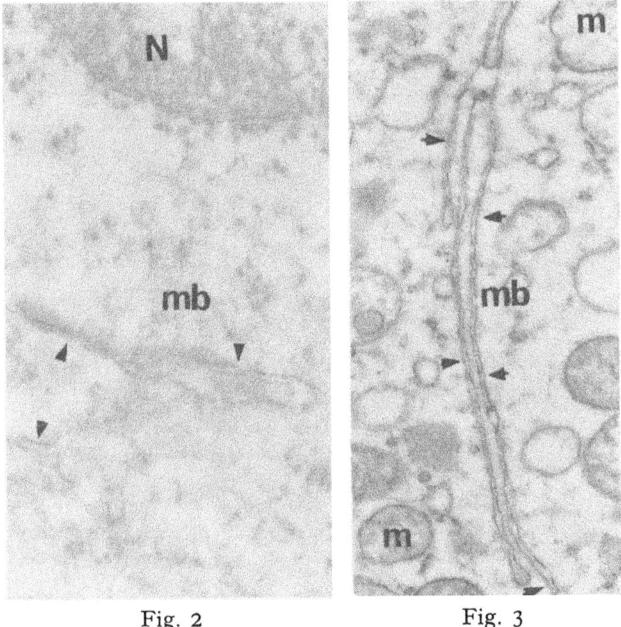

Fig. 2   Fig. 3

Fig. 2. Portion of giant cell showing remnants of folded cytoplasmic membranes (*mb*). × 33 000. Azar and Lunardelli (1969), with permission of the publishers

Fig. 3. Portion of giant cell with paired segments of cytoplasmic membrane (*mb*). × 33 000. Azar and Lunardelli (1969), with permission of the publishers

undergo *in vitro* blastogenesis prior to mitotic division. It has also been shown that such transformed lymphocytes may continue after 48 to 72 hours to develop the morphologic features of large histiocytes or macrophages (Okano *et al.*, 1968).

An alternative hypothesis to the origin of epithelioid cells from circulating lymphocytes and mononuclear cells is that they arise from local reticuloendothelial cells. Such a hypothesis does not, however, explain the frequently widespread and systemic nature of sarcoidosis, its relationship to blood vessels, and its avoidance of the central nervous system. Even this hypothesis needs to go further as to explain the ancestry of reticuloendothelial cells.

Among the experimental means of inducing epithelioid granulomas, metal-induced granulomas in man offer a particularly useful model for the study of

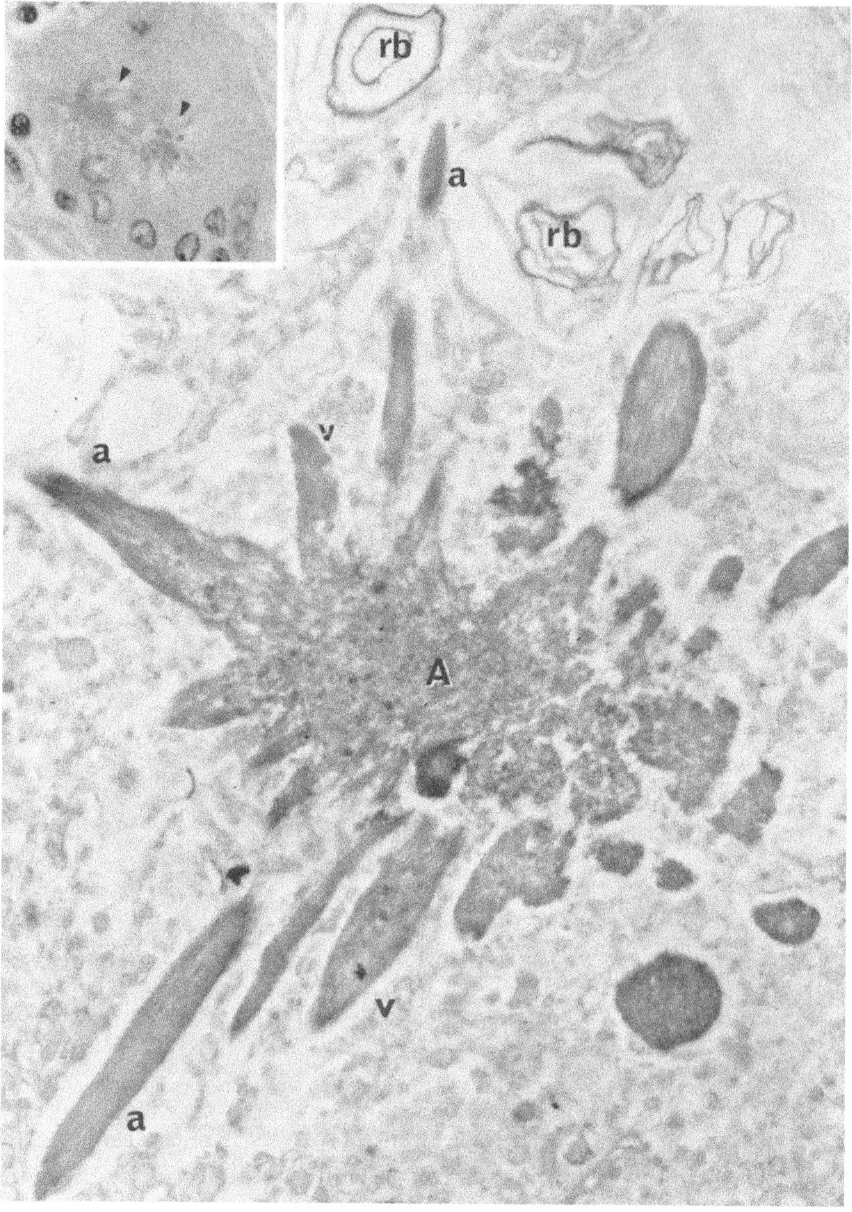

Fig. 4. Asteroid body (*A*) with multiple peripheral arms (*a*). Note also vesicles (*v*) and concentric residual bodies (*rb*). × 10800. Insert demonstrate light microscopic appearance of asteroid bodies in a giant cell. H & E. × 400. Azar and Lunardelli (1969), with permission of the publishers

the derivation of epithelioid cells. Ultrastructural studies of these granulomas have suggested that epithelioid cells do not evolve from phagocytes containing the metals but from undifferentiated mononuclear cells. In individuals sensitized to zirconium and beryllium, epithelioid cells seem to develop from mononuclear

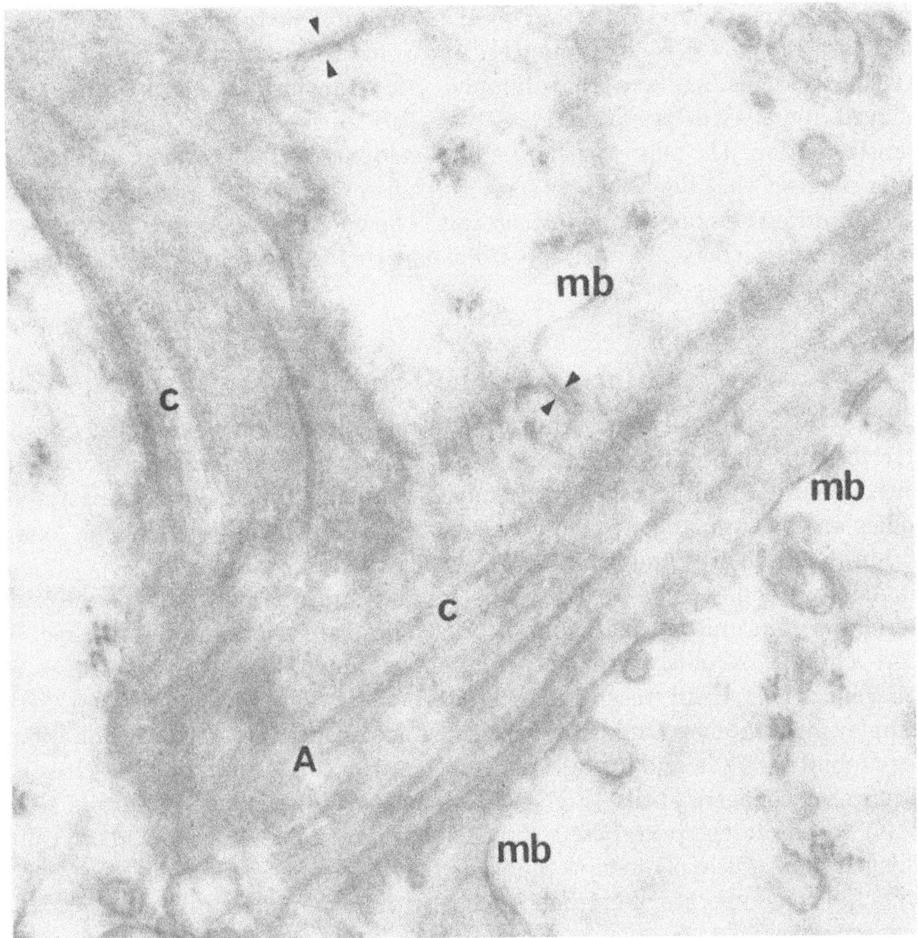

Fig. 5. Two arms of asteroid body (*A*) with fibers showing the 640–700 Å periodicity of collagen (*c*). Note remnants of cytoplasmic membranes (*mb*) suggesting that the formation of asteroid bodies takes place at the site of incomplete fusion of neighboring epithelioid cells. × 66000. AZAR and LUNARDELLI (1969), with permission of the publishers

cells which appeared perivascularly within 2 weeks after intradermal injection of the metal and began to organize into tubercles (ELIAS and EPSTEIN, 1968).

As an extension to the above observations, EPSTEIN and KRASNOBROD (1968) in a study of the origin of epithelioid cells in metal-induced epithelioid granulomas of man, injected at intervals from 4 days to 9 months tritiated thymidine at the site of developing granulomas. Their autoradiographic preparations indicate that a significant number of epithelioid cells in zirconium and beryllium-induced granulomas is derived from medium to large mononuclear cells. This cell is initially distributed in perivascular foci along with lymphocytes and sometimes plasma cells. In earlier lesions, the seemingly blood-borne mononuclear cells appear simply to produce other mononuclear cells. After a critical cell mass has accumulated by influx and mitosis, cells proceed to differentiate and become epithelioid cells that tend to organize in tubercles. This process continues at a slower pace for months. According to Epstein and Krasnobrod (1968), it seems unlikely that lymphocytic transformation, as in *in vitro* delayed hypersensitivity reactions, plays an active role in granulomatous transformation. The close association of developing epithelioid cells to lymphocytes suggests that lymphocytes serve to transmit or receive a message involving the differentiating mononuclear cell. The mononuclear precursor of epithelioid cells seems to be derived from hematogenous sources as is the case for most macrophages.

C. Inclusions and Significance

The two classically important inclusions of multinucleated giant cells described in relation to sarcoidosis but not pathognomonic of this condition since they are found in other granulomas, including tuberculosis, are asteroid bodies and Schaumann's bodies. The two types of inclusions may be found within the same area and occasionally within the same giant cell.

Asteroid bodies may be defined as roughly multipronged, star-shaped inclusions within multinucleated giant cells. These are more likely to be seen in more chronic or older forms of granulomas, undergoing various stages of collagenization. Until recently, asteroid bodies were thought to represent complex lipoproteins. Under the electron microscope, the asteroid formations were found by Azar and Lunardelli (1969) to be constituted by criss-crossing bundles of collagen fibrils (Fig. 4, 5). Some of these collagen deposits were found to be closely juxtaposed to cell membranes and "inside" giant cells. This paradox was explained on the basis that Langhans giant cells represent a syncytial conglomerate of epithelioid cells with incompletely fused cytoplasmic membranes (Fig. 2, 3).

The presence of collagen bundles within giant cells brings the question whether these are part of the ubiquitous collagen found in interstitial spaces, or whether these have been selectively formed in loco by epithelioid cells during the healing stage of granulomas. The latter possibility is favored particularly in view of the findings of McDougal and Azar (1971) that macrophages may be involved in the synthesis of collagen (also see below under subsection E. "Fibrous Healing").

Schaumann's bodies may be defined as concentric, calcified microspherules found either free or in relation to giant cells of sarcoid granulomas, and other granulomatous reactions. These bodies have been studied ultrastructurally in man as well as in experimental conditions (Dumont and Sheldon, 1965). We have already referred to the observation that the epithelioid cell, and also multinucleated giant cells, may contain a considerable number of complex lysosomal granules of autophagic nature. These often coalesce, and undergo mineralization, thus forming the nidus for bigger complexes which are then recognized under the light microscope as Schaumann's bodies (Fig. 5). It would seem, therefore, that both asteroid bodies and Schaumann's bodies represent

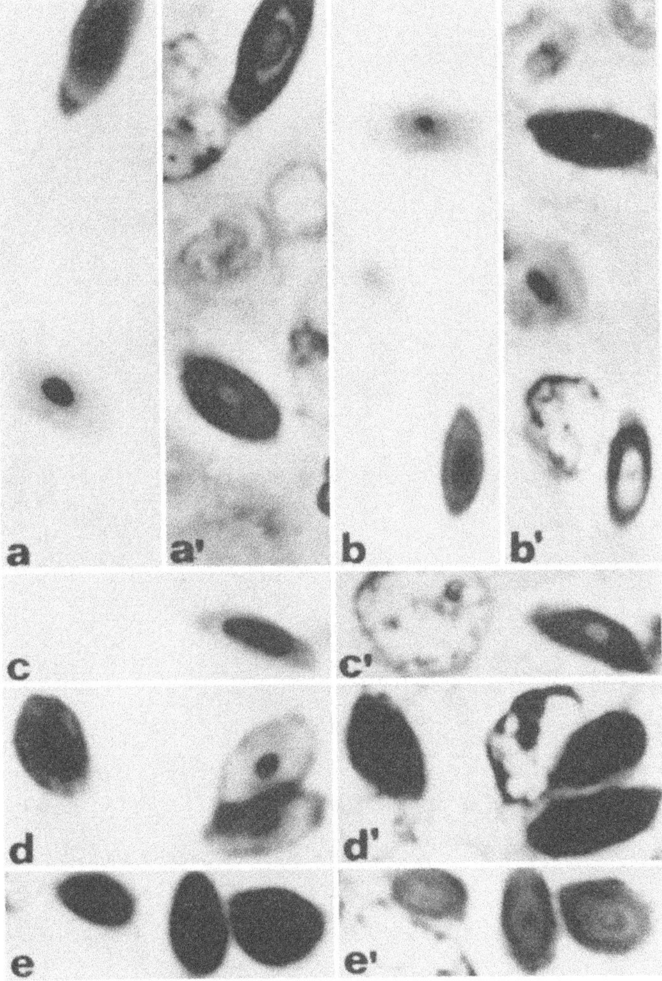

Fig. 6. Light microscope appearance of larger pigment granules (*a–e*) with corresponding phase contrast appearance (*a'–e'*). These are usually seen in reticulo-endothelial cells outside epithelioid granulomas. Note the dense "nucleoids". Iron stain, Lillie. × 800

healing phases of a granuloma: one by collagenization; the second, by auto-phagocytosis.

D. Pigment Granules in Sarcoid Lymph Nodes

This puzzling and highly controversial subject has been debated for decades, and revived recently by CARTER and GROSS (1969). In summary, paraffin sections of formalin-fixed tissue of human lymph nodes harboring sarcoid lesions frequently contain minute, lightly-pigmented bodies measuring from 2.0 to 20 micra in diameter. These are stainable with Schiff's reagent in acid pH of 3.0 to 3.5, and exhibit a variable degree of positivity for stainable iron (Fig. 6). Under the electron microscope, these granules appear as membrane-

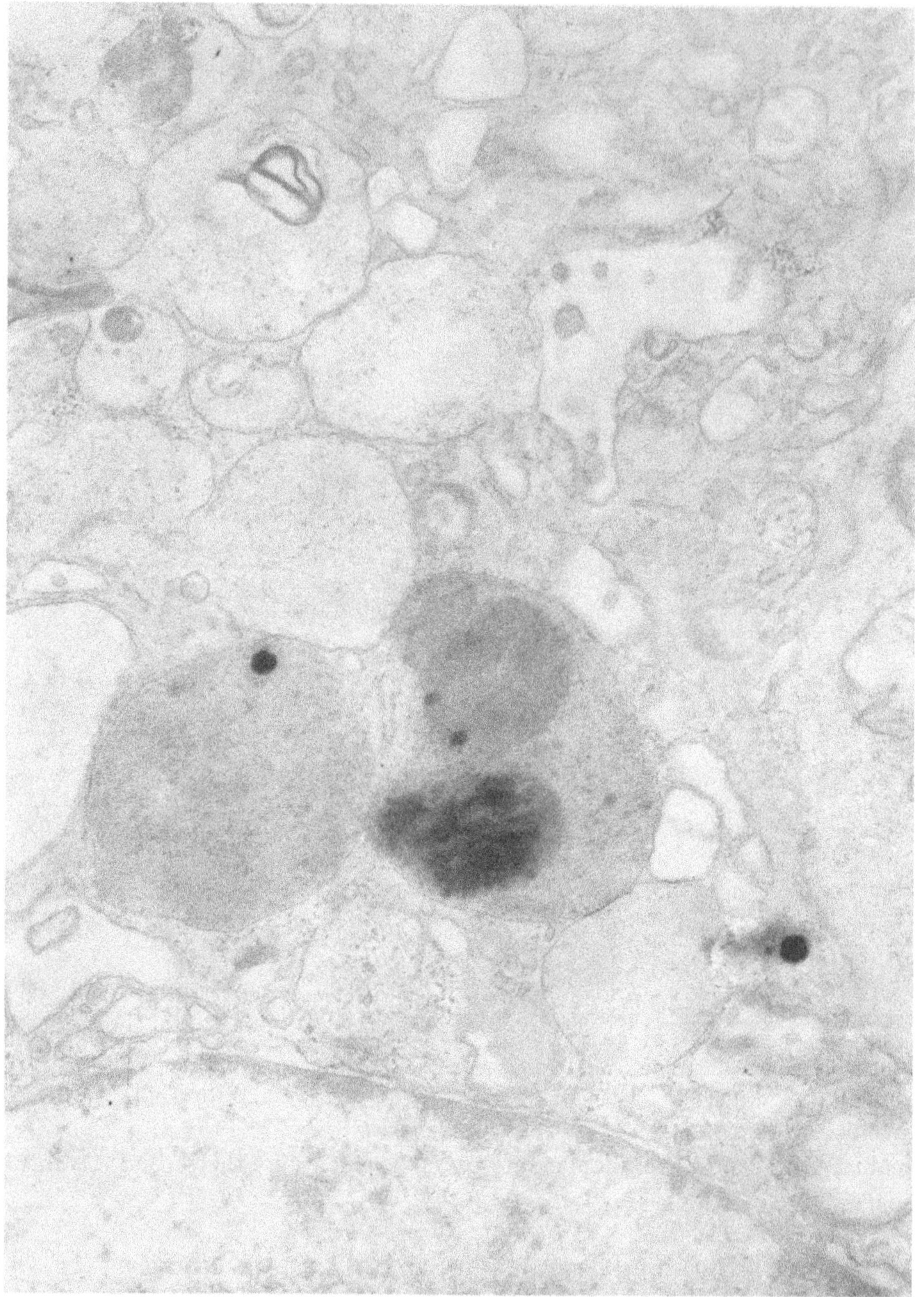

Fig. 7. Confluent pigment granules with "nucleoids" in various stages of development.
× 39000

bound structures with varying density, often containing one to several dense "nucleoids" in various stages of development, as well as free smaller dense granules (Fig. 7). In many instances, the granules resemble phagolysosomes.

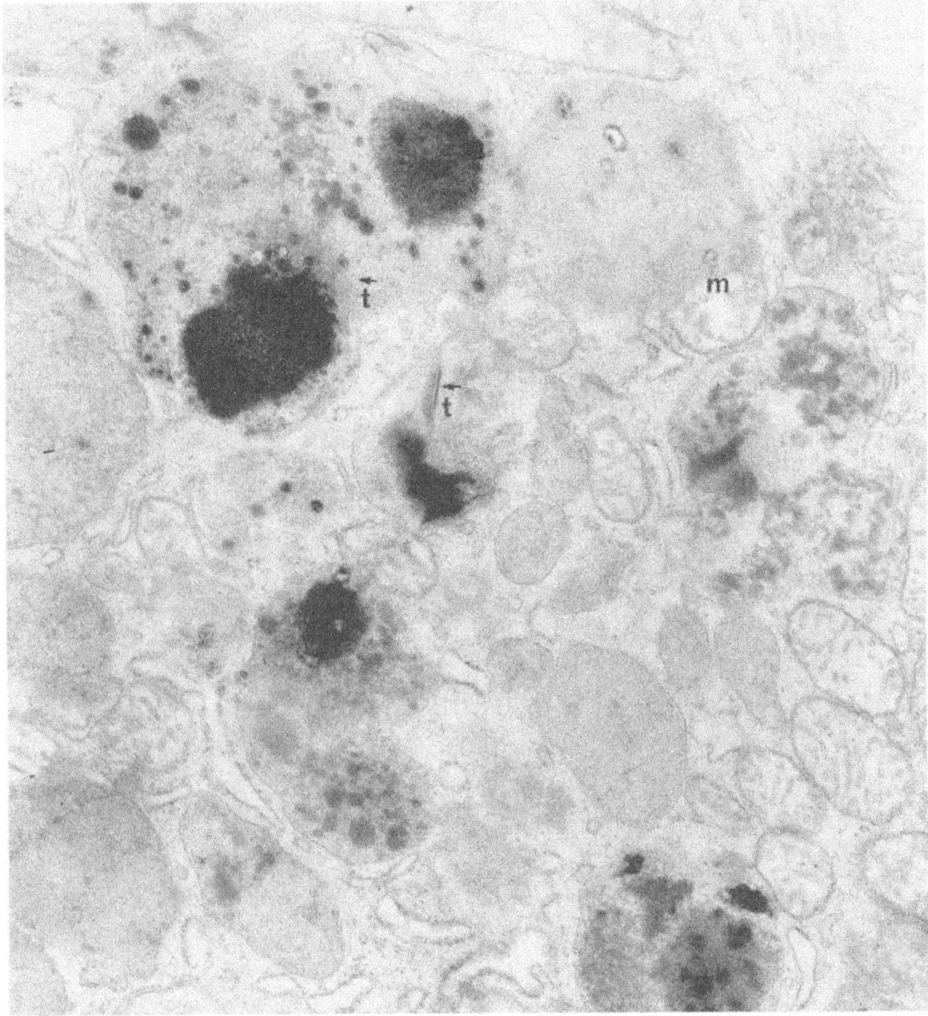

Fig. 8. Pigment granules in various stages of development, some resembling complex phagolysomes, incorporating a mitochondrion (m) or tubular processes (t). $\times 39\,000$

Occasionally, one can see evidence of autophagic activity with incorporation of a fragment of degenerating mitochondrion (Fig. 8), or of concentric lamellae or folded myelin formations (Fig. 9).

It must be emphasized that the pigment granules are not as a rule present within the epithelioid granulomas themselves. They are more likely to be present in the peripheral sinusoids among reticuloendothelial cells outside the epithelioid aggregates. Smaller, one-micron wide, "residual bodies" have been repeatedly observed in epithelioid cells and giant cells of various forms of granulomatous inflammation (WILLIAMS and WILLIAMS, 1967). Even smaller, lipoid or ceroid-like pigments have been described by KALKOFF and HOLTZ (1964) in sarcoidosis and other granulomas.

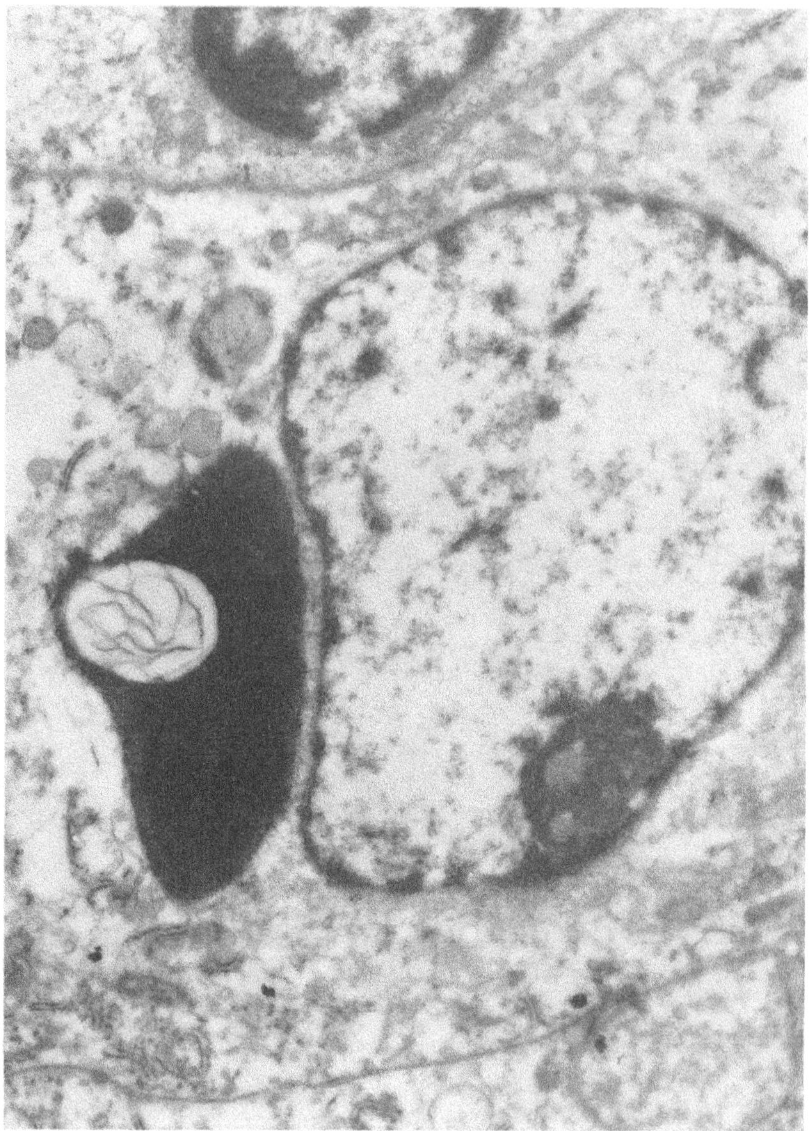

Fig. 9. Pigment granule with incorporation of folded "myelin" formations. × 39000

As to the interpretation of the larger pigment granules seen almost exclusively in sarcoid lymph nodes but outside the granulomas proper, these have been considered to be atypical mycobacterial forms, yeasts, or, according to Moscovic and Neptune (1969), protozoan-like structures.

More recently, Moscovic (1971) studied in detail the histochemical reactions of the pigment granules of sarcoid lymph nodes ("Hamazaki granules") and, while recognizing that they gave most of the characteristic reactions of ceroid-lipofuscin group of pigments, he concluded these granules differed from any endogenous pigments by their unusually low isoelectric point and high phospholipid contrast. Observing that these granules occurred in distinct "spindle forms", "ring forms", "bleb forms" and "round forms", with morphologic details *sui generis* such as "nucleoids", refractile vacuoles and granules and evidence of budding. MOSCOVIC concluded that this high level of organization suggested developmental forms of an unknown organism, or group of related organisms.

Although a comprehensive study of nucleic acids using the Feulgen reaction, basic dyes and induced fluorescence with acridine orange with or without hydrolysis failed to show conclusively that DNA is present in the pigment granules, this study seemed to reveal a highly basophilic and poorly hydrolyzable form of RNA invariably distributed at the periphery of the granules. In addition, acridine orange-stained granules showed the same rim fluorescence that has been described in relation to various fluorochromes as characteristic of large bodies of Mycoplasma and bacterial L-forms (KANG and CASIDA, 1967). While these reactions by themselves were considered by MOSCOVIC to be highly suggestive of bacterial L-forms, it was furthermore noted that some of the smaller granules within the pigment granules gave the characteristic phase contrast and histochemical reaction of volutin granules or inorganic polyphosphates (HAROLD, 1966). Since volutin granules are commonly found in the exponential phase of bacterial growth under adverse nutritional conditions, and do not occur in organisms above the subkingdom of *Thallophyta*, MOSCOVIC assumes that the pigment granules of sarcoid lymph nodes are of exogenous origin and concludes that these granules represent viable bacterial L-forms.

An alternative hypothesis based on the ultrastructural study of pigment granules of sarcoid lymph nodes (AZAR *et al.*, 1970) is that these granules represent the end product of incomplete or inadequate autophagic digestion within complex lysosomal bodies or autophagosomes. In other words, these granules probably represent structures analogous to the lipofuscin pigments seen in the senile heart (MALKOFF and STREHLER, 1963), in the liver (ESSNER and NOVIKOFF, 1960), and sometimes in smooth muscle of viscera of aging or chronically ill patients.

Why do sarcoid lymph nodes harbor large pigment granules in abundance? The obvious answer, should their origin be ascribed to lysosomal granules, would be that there may be an enzymatic defect in the reticuloendothelial system of sarcoid patients resulting in the accumulation of products of incomplete digestion or residual bodies. The pigment granules may represent, therefore, the storage of undigested phagocytosed material without reference to whether this material is of exogenous origin, or to whether it is entirely a product of autophagic activity. It must be also pointed out that the Kveim granulomas do not harbor large pigment granules. This is anticipated in view of the fact that the Kveim reaction represents the products of a four to six-week lesion, whereas the large pigment granules found in sarcoid lymph nodes have been probably accumulated over months or years.

E. Fibrous Healing

The relatively benign nature of sarcoid lesions has long been recognized. Sarcoid lesions are often self-healing. With the introduction of steroid therapy, one can readily witness their rapid disappearance. We have, on

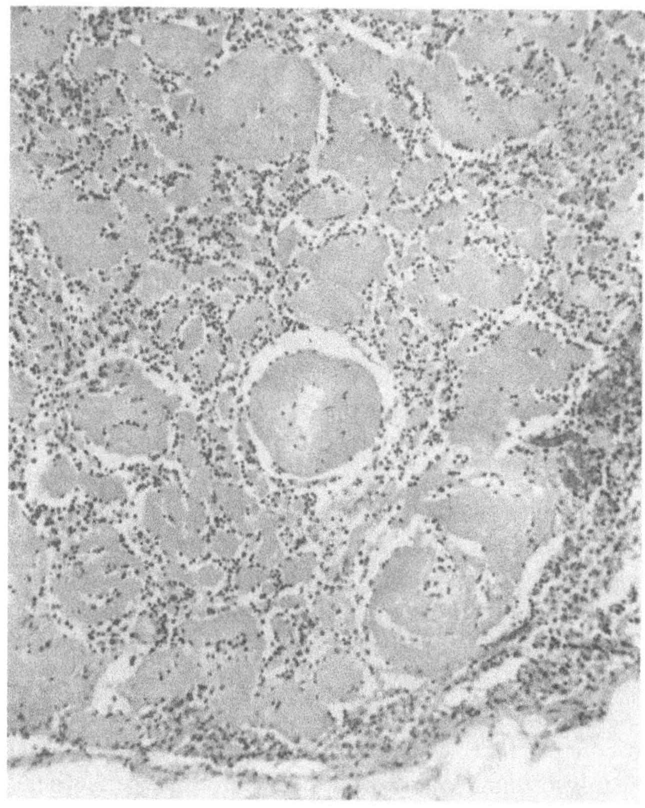

Fig. 10. Hyalinized nodules in a lymph node maintaining the overall architecture of a sarcoid-type granulomatous reaction. H & E, × 110

occasion, examined sections of sarcoid lesions after prolonged treatment with corticosteroids, and been impressed by the amount of collagenization present in areas formerly occupied by epithelioid granulomas (Fig. 10).

Since epithelial granulomas heal so readily by fibrosis, and because of the possibility that asteroid bodies are laid down in loco by epithelioid cells transforming into fibroblasts, McDougal and Azar (1971) investigated the possibility of such a transformation by testing the ability of macrophages of foreign-body granulomas to metabolize tritiated proline and release it in relation to the intercellular connective tissue matrix. In autoradiographic analysis of such tissues, it was possible to demonstrate that immediately following *in vivo* injection of a pulse of tritiated proline, or of an *in vitro* incubation with the same agent, the macrophages of a talcum or mycobacterial granuloma incorporate the label within the cytoplasm, and tend to release it within 24 hours in the matrix. This is illustrated in Figs. 11 and 12. It is obvious, therefore, that we are dealing here with a fluid situation where there may be a series of cellular metamorphoses beginning with blood-borne mononuclear cells to collagen-forming cells via epithelioid cells.

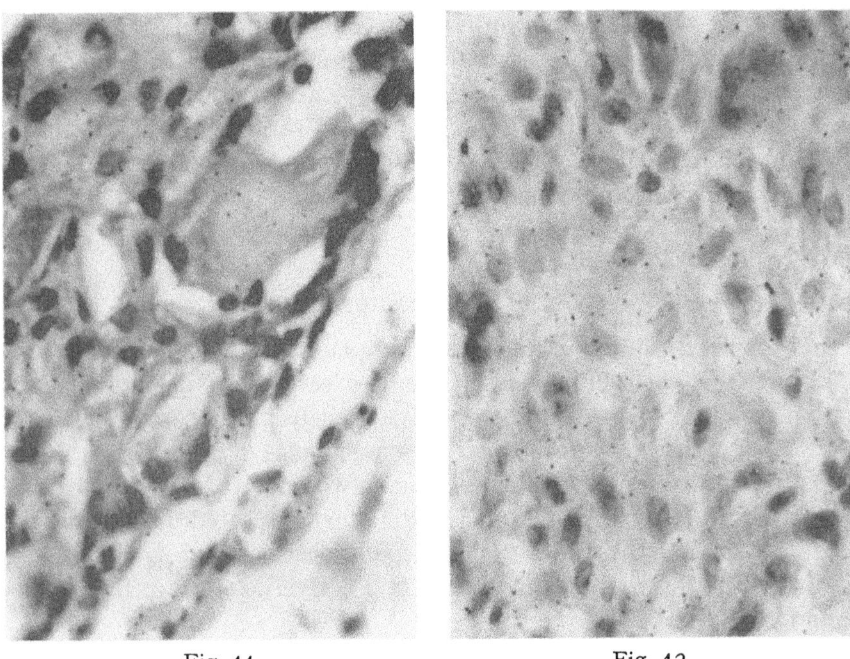

Fig. 11   Fig. 12

Fig. 11. Tritiated proline label in cytoplasm of macrophages of talcum granuloma, 2 hours after injection of the label. H & E, × 624. McDougal and Azar (1971), with permission of the publishers

Fig. 12. Tritiated proline label scattered both within and outside cytoplasmic fields of macrophages of talcum granuloma, 24 hours after injection of the label. H & E, × 624. McDougal and Azar (1971) with permission of the publishers

The ultrastructure of the hyalin changes in sarcoidosis has been studied by Gusek (1968) and by Kalifat et al. (1969). In addition to collagen, it has been suggested that the ground substance of sarcoid granuloma contains a "hyalin" substance, "fibrinoid" as well as "paramyloid". Unfortunately, these three terms are vague inasmuch as they cannot be translated into any precise biochemical or morphological constituent. The use of the term "paramyloid" is particularly misleading since the various amyloid deposits were all shown to have the same histochemical and ultrastructural characteristics (Azar, 1968). There is no evidence known to us that sarcoidosis predisposes in any significant manner to localized or systemic amyloidosis.

III. Review of Etiological Factors

One of the classical approaches in the study of sarcoidosis is that this condition, despite its many clinical variations, could be ascribed to one specific etiologic factor. Obviously, the past century has seen a number of clinico-pathological syndromes become, one by one, linked to a specific causative factor be it a genetic defect, a microorganism, a virus or a chemical. The search for a causative agent in sarcoidosis did not seem, therefore, to be illogical. Because of the great resemblance between the lesions of sarcoidosis, and those of tuberculosis, the first attempt to search for an etiologic agent centered around mycobacteria, including attenuated, or atypical forms of these organisms. Indeed, there is evidence that tuberculous and sarcoid lesions may co-exist in the same individual; as the signs and symptoms of one condition abate, those of the other become unmasked (Haroutunian *et al.*, 1964).

A. Mycobacteria

From the very beginning, there were arguments for and against the acceptance of the tubercle bacillus as the agent of sarcoidosis despite the lack of caseation and absence of demonstrable acid-fast bacilli in sarcoid lesions, and the difficulty of growing mycobacteria from samples of such lesions. Furthermore, it became apparent soon that patients with sarcoidosis did not respond with the usual tuberculin test in the manner expected from tuberculous patients. In spite of these reservations, the hypothesis that sarcoidosis represents an unusual form of tuberculosis is still actively entertained (Siltzbach, 1968 and 1969).

The possible role of atypical mycobacteria as an etiologic factor in sarcoidosis has been explored by Mankiewicz (1963) who reported the isolation of bacteriophages lytic for tubercle bacilli in both tuberculous patients and patients with sarcoidosis. While tuberculous patients were found to have phage-neutralizing antibodies, patients with sarcoidosis did not. *In vitro* experiments showed that in the absence of neutralizing antibodies, phagolysis and lysogenic conversion of tubercle bacilli took place. The end result of lysogeny was the emergence of bacilli so modified in their antigenic and morphological appearance, including acid-fastness, that they could no longer be recognized as tubercle bacilli. From six lymph nodes obtained from patients with sarcoidosis and cultured in a variety of media, including media containing anti-phage sera, five variant strains of tubercle bacilli were isolated. Mankiewicz concluded that the above observations support the view that certain cases of sarcoidosis are due to "modified" tubercle bacilli.

More recently, Bowman (1968) studied 70 sera from different patients with sarcoidosis. Serum neutralization activity could be demonstrated in 91 to 98 % against mycobacteriophages D29, Leo or R1. Of 81 sera from non-sarcoid patients, neutralizing activity was demonstrated in 83 to 85 % against phages D29 and Leo, and in 100 % against phages R1. In tests using phage R1, the magnitude of K values of sera of patients not having sarcoidosis was much larger than those of patients with sarcoidosis. This interesting observation of the failure of patients with sarcoidosis to produce R1 antibodies remains to be explained. BOWMAN also notes that *M. butyricum* is naturally lysogenic with phage R1, and is ubiquitously distributed in nature.

CHAPMAN and SPEIGHT (1964) studied the sera of 280 patients with sarcoidosis and detected precipitin antibody reactions to mycobacterial agents in 79.7 % of these sera. Sera from 770 control cases have been studied with the more reactive mycobacterial antigens and 31 % of the control sera showed significant reactions. The antigens used comprised photochromagens, scotochromogens, non-chromagens, and mixed "non-pathogens". Sarcoidosis could not be related specifically to any atypical or unclassified mycobacterium. Members of all three of Runyon's group were represented among the reacting strains.

More recently, VANĚK and SCHWARZ (1970) studied 30 consecutive cases of sarcoidosis, and found acid-fast bacilli in every instance on microscopic examination. The acid-fast bacilli were seen either as isolated bacilli, or in groups. An effort to photograph these structures met with considerable difficulty; however, in their three illustrations, the acid-fast bacilli appeared to be quite distinct. It is obvious that a prolonged search was devoted to the finding of these isolated mycobacteria. The authors' material being in great part retrospective, culture was possible only in isolated instances. They also admit that only in the relatively rare cases of sarcoidosis in which acid- fast bacilli were cultivated and classified, have the human, bovine, avian or anonymous types of tubercle bacilli been identified.

In our own experience (see WILNER et al., 1969) with a study of paraffin sections of tuberculous and sarcoid granulomas stained with auramine and rhodamine and viewed with the fluorescence microscope, beaded yellow-orange fluorescent mycobacterial forms were found in 10 of 16 cases of tuberculous lesions. No such organisms could be identified in any of the sections of lymph nodes obtained from 42 patients with sarcoidosis of two different geographical locations (27 cases from Beirut, and 15 cases from New York). Mycobacterial forms were not observed in Kveim granulomas. In view of our repeated failure to recognize mycobacteria or mycobacterial fragments in sarcoid granulomas by such means as fluorescence or electron microscopy, it has become increasingly difficult to readily accept a concept based on the mycobacterial etiology of sarcoidosis, even if the incriminated mycobacteria were atypical or in the process of being phage-lysed.

B. Pollen

CUMMINGS et al. (1956) reported that the distribution of sarcoidosis was similar to that of pine trees, both predominating in the Southeastern United States. The communities with the highest prevalence rates had lumbering and forest products as principal industries. Sarcoidosis was particularly prevalent among Negroes. This interesting observation was not borne out, however, in several epidemiological surveys. A significant correlation between sarcoidosis and exposure to pine is particularly not borne out in European surveys (HALL et al., 1969). In spite of this lack of correlation with exposure to conifers, the findings of Cummings may still be valid for the Southern United States and should deserve attention in view of experimental data showing that instillation of pine extracts in the respiratory tree lead to the formation of pulmonary granulomas mimicking those of sarcoidosis.

VOGEL (1967) instilled pine pollen in guinea pigs and mice and produced granulomas constituted by epithelioid cells, some Langhans giant cells and occasional amorphous calcific inclusions. These lesions did not, however, contain as many epithelioid cells as the sarcoid granulomas of man. VOGEL's serological studies on patients did not establish any obvious correlation between sarcoidosis and mycobacterial antibodies, but revealed an apparent suppression of circulating antibody to pine pollen at the time of maximal pollen concentration in the environment. VOGEL also notes that the greatest number of cases of sarcoidosis recorded in a North Carolina institution are observed during the months of March, April and May which are also the months of maximal shedding of pollen not only from pine, but from other varieties of trees.

C. Other Agents

Exposures to various dusts of mineral, vegetable or animal sources, even clay-eating, and social factors, have all been investigated as possible etiological factors in sarcoidosis (HALL et al., 1969).

In addition to mycobacteria, a number of microorganisms have been also historically linked with sarcoidosis. Among these, one may cite *Mycobacterium leprae*, *Treponema pallidum*, *Brucella* organisms, and viruses. Recently, HIRSHAUT et al. (1970) investigated the association of herpes-like virus and sarcoidosis. The herpes-like virus was detected in lymphoid cell cultures derived from Burkitt tumor, and has been suggested as the etiologic agent of infectious mononucleosis. It has also been suspected of playing a part in the pathogenesis of both the African Burkitt lymphoma and carcinoma of the posterior nasal space. The study of HIRSHAUT et al., deals with sera from 131 patients with sarcoidosis. All had antibody to herpes-like virus, and in 79% the titers were 1/640 or higher. This contrasted with a 76% prevalence of antibody in a control group with considerably lower titers. Since four diseases, including sarcoidosis have been associated with the herpes-like virus, the authors emphasize that any conclusions regarding the pathogenic role of this virus in any given condition must be made cautiously. The unequivocal assignment of herpes-like virus to a disease entity must ultimately depend on the induction of this disease in a suitable animal host with purified herpes-like virus. Of course, the possibility of a special susceptibility of patients with sarcoidosis to herpes-like virus is of note and deserves further investigation.

D. A Specific but Hitherto Undiscovered Agent or a Miscellany of Trivial Agents?

Of course, the frustration that has accompanied so far the search for an etiologic agent in sarcoidosis need not necessarily denote that such an agent does not exist. Similar frustrations have accompanied the current search for an agent in a variety of diseases thought to be caused by an infectious agent. Among these, one may list infectious and serum hepatitis, Aleutian-mink disease, periodic disease or familial Mediterranean fever, etc. As more specific infectious, or non-infectious agents become incriminated in various granulomas, the hard-core residuum may continue to constitute what we call sarcoidosis. This residuum, of course, may be due to one or several agents that remain to be unmasked.

It is equally possible that sarcoidosis may not represent a lesion due to a specific etiologic factor, but a form of host reaction to miscellaneous, trivial, indigenous, or exogenous agents. In other words, sarcoidosis may be analogous to keloidal scarring which often develops as a result of trivial trauma. It is the underlying genetic make-up of the individual with keloids which is of greater importance than the factor of trauma per se. This approach to the understanding of sarcoidosis is becoming increasingly attractive, particularly to the immunologist, or immunology-oriented pathologist, and will be given more consideration below.

IV. The Kveim Reaction

Since neither the clinical nor the histologic manifestation of sarcoidosis are pathognomonic, there arose a need for a more objective test for sarcoidosis to differentiate this condition from other granulomatous conditions of known etiology: tuberculosis, leprosy, histoplasmosis, brucellosis, and berylliosis, among others.

The Nickerson-Kveim test more recently standardized and tested in an international study (SILTZBACH, 1967) consists of the intracutaneous administration of a test dose of a suspension derived from a human sarcoidal spleen. The test site is examined at 6 weeks, and punch biopsies of the skin are performed if any macular or papular lesions were discernible. A "positive" test results in a histological picture of non-necrotizing granuloma which bears a striking resemblance to sarcoid-type lesions.

A. Positive and "Negative" Reactions

The international Kveim test study of 1960–1966, headed by SILTZBACH (1967) and carried out with the Chase-Siltzbach "Type 1" suspension derived from a single human sarcoidal spleen, was conducted in 37 countries. The patients tested belonged to 3 categories: Group 1, biopsy-confirmed sarcoidosis; Group 2, sarcoidosis suspects; Group 3, controls. The histological picture of positive papular lesions obtained from all these countries was similar. This led Siltzbach to lean toward a hypothesis that sarcoidosis is a single distinct disorder. There were, however, marked variations in the percentage of positive Kveim responses from country to country even in Group 1 subacute cases (96% in Finland, 23% in Germany). False positive Kveim reactions were found in only 0.7% controls, mostly in Japanese patients who had leprosy. It is interesting that in this vast international study comprising over 2,000 biopsy specimens, there is no mention of biopsy of "negative" or non-papular sites of injection.

Enthusiastic reports regarding the potency and specificity of the Kveim reaction continue to appear (James et al., 1969; Celikoglu and Siltzbach, 1969). The percentage of positive reactions was considerably greater in patients with active and disseminated disease than in chronic or localized sarcoidosis. False positive tests with the Chase-Siltzbach preparation seem to have been infrequent. A recent evaluation by Israel and Goldstein (1971) of Kveim tests in 37 selected patients with sarcoidosis revealed that a reaction could be related to persistent lymphadenopathy, and not to duration or activity of illness. Fourteen asymptomatic patients with marked enlargement of the mediastinal and hilar lymph nodes of long duration all reacted strongly. Positive tests occurred in only 3 of 12 patients having disease of recent onset with minimal adenopathy; in only one of 11 with active hepatic or cutaneous sarcoidosis and normal chest roentgenograms. Typical reactions were obtained in patients with chronic lymphocytic leukemia, tuberculous adenitis, infectious mononucleosis, and non-specific cervical adenitis. The authors conclude that the Kveim test appears to be an immunologic reaction associated with persistent lymphadenopathy of diverse causes, rather than a specific reaction of sarcoidosis alone.

B. Morphological Aspects

The resemblance of the Kveim granuloma to that of the parent sarcoid granuloma is striking. The essential features of a non-caseating granuloma are found here. Early during the testing, one can see histiocytic cells phagocytosing cell debris. Later on, at four weeks, after injection of the Kveim reagent and beyond, the granulomas become strikingly epithelioid (Fig. 13, 14). As a rule, no Schaumann's bodies are present. Occasional asteroid bodies may be observed within Langhans-type giant cells. No pigment granules are present at the periphery of the Kveim granuloma. Lymphocytes, plasma cells and mononuclear cells may be seen in the general area of the injection, and in between epithelioid granulomas. The ultrastructure of the epithelioid cells in the Kveim granuloma is strikingly similar to that in sarcoid epithelioid cells (Hirsch et al., 1967). It must be emphasized that the positivity to the Kveim reaction is a matter of degree, and that even clinically negative individuals, i.e. individuals who fail to show a nodule approximately four weeks after injection of the antigen, have actually, on microscopic examination of the injection site, a minor epithelioid or foreign-body type reaction. The division between negative and positive Kveim reaction can be, in our experience, a very arbitrary matter. This is easier to settle clinically, on the basis of palpation, rather than histologically. For our purposes, we would consider the matter of Kveim reactivity as a matter of degree, rather than an all or none phenomenon.

C. The Active Component of the Kveim Reagent

Since the Kveim reagent, including the Chase-Siltzbach preparation, is a coarse suspension of homogenized sarcoid tissue which has been heat-sterilized and kept under asceptic conditions, it is interesting to speculate about the component of this suspension which is responsible for the production of the granulomatous reaction.

The only serious attempt to analyze the component of the Kveim reaction as to the factor responsible for the induction of the granuloma is that carried out by COHN and his associates (1967). Lymph nodes obtained from active cases of sarcoidosis were homogenized, and subcellular fractions obtained by differential and gradient centrifugation. The reactivity of various fractions was assayed by intradermal injections into Kveim positive and negative patients. Most of the material with Kveim activity appeared at centrifugal forces below 15,000 g. In sucrose gradients, Kveim activity was associated with cytoplasmic particles which equilibrated between 50 and 70 percent sucrose. By electron microscopy, and acid phosphatase assays of the subcellular fractions, it was apparent that the Kveim activity was localized to membrane-bound dense bodies, probably of lysosomal nature. COHN *et al.* speculated that since dense bodies arise by means of either pinocytosis or phagocytosis, they may contain soluble macromolecules or particulate components of their environment. The material with Kveim activity may be the particle segregated within dense bodies. The nature of the precise lysosomal component with Kveim reactivity remains to be determined.

D. *In vitro* Kveim Reaction

In vitro systems for an estimation of a specific immunologic reactivity of lymphocytes and dependent on their ability to transform into blast cells in the presence of the specific antigen, have been used in a variety of situations. This method was employed using Kveim antigen as the provoking agent. Unfortunately, little progress has been achieved in this field. This maybe partly due to the difficulties of maintaining lymphocytes in culture for 6 to 8 days.

The antigen-induced inhibition of the *in vitro* migration of macrophages has been used as a parameter of cellular hypersensitivity. This reaction has been adopted for use in man in various hypersensitivity states. HARDT and WANSTRUP (1969) have adopted this test in a sarcoidosis antigen system. Their material consisted of seven patients with sarcoidosis verified by biopsy in various stages of development, and six patients with active tuberculous

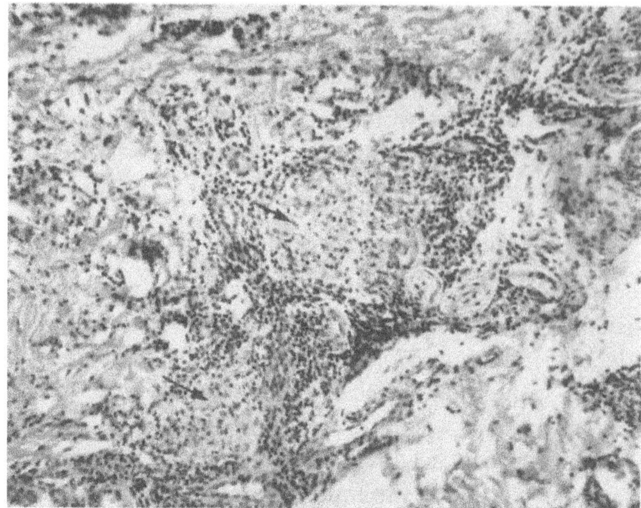

Fig. 13. Biopsy site of clinically negative Kveim reaction. Note (arrows) diminutive epithelioid granulomas. H & E, × 110

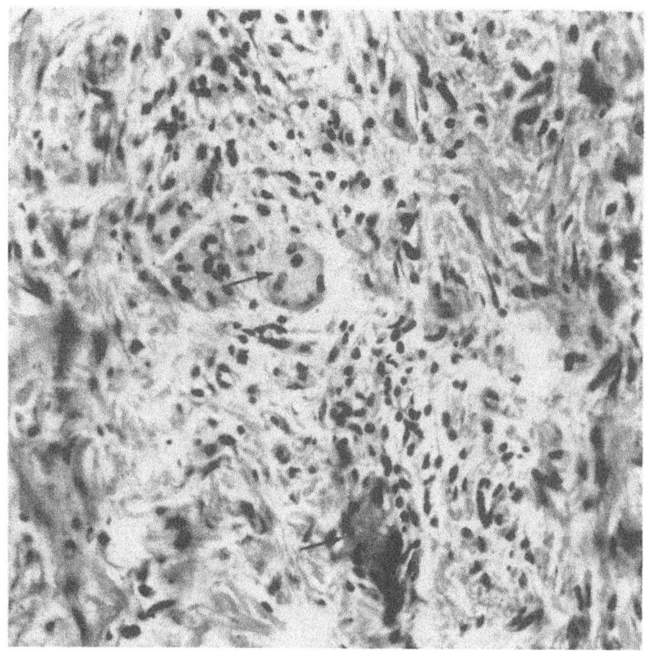

Fig. 14. Biopsy site of clinically negative Kveim reaction. Note (arrows) multinucleated giant cell in field of mixed histiocytic and lymphocytic reaction. H & E, × 110

infections. Control groups comprised 9 healthy persons. Peripheral leukocytes were isolated, and placed in capillary tubes. The tubes were then placed in a culture chamber containing nutrient medium. 150 µg of Kveim antigen, measured by protein content was added to half the number of chambers.

As the Kveim antigen is preserved with phenol, the suspension was dialyzed against Hank's balanced salt solution for 48 hours. The migration areas were measured 24 hours later by paper planimetry. Migration index was calculated in the following way: migration in chambers containing antigen/migration in chambers without antigen. Thus, the migration index indicates an inhibition of the cell migration if these values are lower than 1, and a stimulation, if the values are greater than 1. All the leucocytes derived from sarcoid patients showed considerable inhibition of their migration *in vitro* when incubated with the Kveim antigen. In contrast, the control cultures from healthy or tuberculous patients showed no, or only very slight, inhibition. These results support the diagnostic relavance of this *in vitro* Kveim system, as leukocytes from sarcoid patients invariably showed pronounced inhibition. It was thus possible in 24 hours to obtain the same information as from the *in vivo* intracutaneous Kveim test which demands 6 to 10 weeks. The authors recognize that larger materials are necessary, and that a comparative study of *in vitro* and *in vivo* Kveim systems is desirable.

E. Biological Significance

Since repeated epidemiological studies (JAMES *et al.*, 1969; CELIGOKLU *et al.*, 1969) have shown the pragmatic value of the *in vivo* Kveim test, it is obvious that we are dealing here with an important biological phenomenon that remains to be interpreted. The Kveim suspension, obviously, does not contain any harmful, infectious agent to normal individuals. If a pathogenic microorganism were to be found in the Kveim suspension, it is obvious that normal and non-sarcoid individuals seem to dispose of it effectively. It is also doubtful that we are dealing here with a minute amount of exogenous chemical which is carried over from the donor of the Kveim reagent into the recipients of Kveim test doses.

We have already alluded to the possibility that no truly negative Kveim reaction exists, as gauged by microscopic criteria (Fig. 13). Since the Kveim reactive material seems to be localized to membrane-bound dense bodies which may be lysosomal in nature (COHN *et al.*, 1967), it is safe to assume that the sarcoid individual as opposed to the non-sarcoid one is unable to properly dispose of this responsible component, and over-reacts to it by the formation of epithelioid granulomas.

As to the gravest pitfalls in Kveim testing, these may be listed as:

1. The difficulty in defining a histologically-negative Kveim reagent.

2. The possibility of false positive reaction due to the presence of non-specific mediastinal and cervical lymphadenopathy (ISRAEL and GOLDSTEIN, 1971).

3. The negative Kveim reactions in localized sarcoidal reaction, particularly in cutaneous sarcoidosis.

In spite of all these pitfalls, the Kveim reagent is a useful diagnostic tool in both *in vivo* and *in vitro* testing of patients with generalized lymphadeno-pathy including those with sarcoidosis.

V. Immunology of Sarcoidosis

Pathologists may need to be reminded that sarcoidosis is not only a morpho-logic reaction and a clinical syndrome, but also, an immunological disorder often characterized by profound alterations in serum immunoglobulins, as well as in delayed hypersensitivity reactions. In addition, there is the more recent appreciation that peripheral lymphocytes of patients with sarcoidosis often show functional aberrations that may have a direct bearing on the sarcoid phenomenon.

A. Immunoglobulins

A diffuse or polyclonal form of hyperglobulinemia is frequently observed in patients with sarcoidosis. Recently, Buckley *et al.* (1970) studied changes in the three major immunoglobulins in patients with sarcoidosis, and tuber-culosis, with respect to age, race, and sex. IgG and IgM were found to be increased in patients with sarcoidosis; IgG in patients with tuberculosis. Differences between serum immunoglobulin concentrations in patients with sarcoidosis and tuberculosis were not significant. In patients with sarcoidosis, the increase in IgG was found to be significant in white patients, and the increase in IgM was significant only in black patients. A similar race-asso-ciated pattern could be demonstrated in patients with tuberculosis. As to sex differences, the increase in IgM in sarcoidosis was only significant in black women. The failure to demonstrate significant differences between serum immunoglobulin concentrations in patients with sarcoidosis and tuberculosis suggests that such determinations cannot provide a basis for distinguishing between the two types of patients.

Daddi (1968) has observed in 75 subjects with sarcoidosis a modest ele-vation in IgA and IgM as compared to a more marked elevation of IgA in tuberculosis, in chronic asthmatic bronchitis, and cirrhosis. The concentration of IgM in patients with sarcoidosis was slightly above the mean of IgM con-centration in tuberculous patients. The total gamma globulin level was moderately elevated, and considerably less than the mean of gamma globulin concentration observed in tuberculous patients. Turiaf *et al.* (1968) have likewise noted that the concentration of immunoglobulins is often increased during the course of sarcoidosis. According to them, the immunoglobulins most frequently increased are of the IgM fraction. Increase in IgA was parti-cularly noted at the initial phase of the disease. The increase in the immuno-globulins was seen particularly in patients with negative tuberculin reactions and a positive Kveim test.

As to the humoral form of antibody production, with the exception of the findings of MANKIEWICZ (1963) who initially demonstrated that sarcoid patients lacked neutralizing antibody against mycobacterialphages, it appears that the response of patients with sarcoidosis to various antigens is essentially the same to that observed in normal individuals. GREENWOOD *et al.* (1958) observed that patients with sarcoidosis produced significantly less circulating antitoxin after primary immunization with tetanus toxoid than controls. A normal response to immunization was given by patients who had been immunized some years earlier. It has also been mentioned above that CHAPMAN and SPEIGHT (1964) have demonstrated in the sera of 80 % of sarcoid patients the presence of an antibody to typical mycobacteria. This has not been confirmed by VOGEL (1967). DADDI (1968) demonstrated antibody to mycobacteria in only 27 out of 102 patients with sarcoidosis. In summary, there appears to be no specific impairment in humoral antibody formation in patients with sarcoidosis. Although such patients do show elevations in the three major classes of immunoglobulins, these changes are variable, and do not convey a specific diagnostic value. It is possible that this increase in immunoglobulin levels is the result of the intense plasmacytic response frequently observed at the periphery of sarcoid granulomas and probably directed against products of autodigestion.

WANSTRUP and ELLING (1968) have investigated lymph nodes from 10 cases of generalized sarcoidosis by means of the fluorescent antibody technique. The sarcoid lymph nodes show basically the same findings. In comparison with control sections, the sarcoid nodes exhibited a far more pronounced content of immunoglobulin. These were accumulated in areas in which the morphology was altered, i.e. the proliferating perigranulomatous and perivascular zones, and within the granulomas proper. The fluorescence of the granulomas varied in extension and intensity, indicating different functional stages of granuloma formation. The three human classes of gamma globulins were found in the tissue, but no safe correlation between the presence of any of these gamma globulins and disease activity could be established. The complement component, beta 1-C globulin, was localized in sarcoid tissue at the same site as gamma globulins. More recently, ELLING and WANSTRUP (1969) reported that in addition to IgG, IgA, and IgM they were able to demonstrate by means of an anti-IgD fluorescent conjugate that IgD was also present within the granulomas.

B. Delayed Hypersensitivity Reactions

A diminished skin reactivity of the delayed hypersensitivity type has long been noted in patients with sarcoidosis who have been tested with tuberculin in an effort to exclude the possibility of tuberculosis. Subsequent studies have shown a significant decrease in reactivity to PPD, including a decreased ability to maintain a positive response following BCG vaccination. This anergy to tuberculin products is still considered an important diagnostic test in sarcoidosis.

A defective, delayed hypersensitivity reaction in patients with sarcoidosis is not confined to tuberculin. Lordon *et al.* (1968) tested, as a part of a prospective study, 50 patients with sarcoidosis for their delayed hypersensitivity response to various antigens. Skin tests with a low reaction rate in normal populations such as intermediate strength PPD, coccidioidin and histoplasmin did not show an appreciable difference in patients with sarcoidosis. A generalized hyporeactivity to the more commonly reactive antigens of Trichophyton, mumps, *Candida albicans*, and PPD-2 was demonstrated. When repeated testing was done, on serial evaluations, a variation in this hyporeactivity was noted that directly related to the activity of disease. A significant decrease in reaction rate to these antigens was shown in patients with active disease when compared with patients with inactive disease. Cutaneous reactivity in the latter patients was similar to that of normal populations. Skin anergy, therefore, seems to have a limited diagnostic value but the reaction rate and size of positive reactions do enable a reasonable measurement of disease activity when performed on serial evaluations. According to Lordon *et al.*, the atypical mycobacterial antigens show the more pronounced hyporeactivity and continued to be negative in spite of repeated applications at various stages of disease activity. Turiaf *et al.* (1968) maintained that the anergy for tuberculin in patients with sarcoidosis probably represents an acquired phenomenon that develops at the beginning of the sarcoid state, and disappeared often after healing of the sarcoid process, but may continue in a number of cases after improvement of the condition. This anergy appears to coincide in a great majority of patients with positive Kveim reactivity. In other word, the anergic state seems to be directly linked to the activity and extent of sarcoidosis, which in turn, is also manifested by a positive Kveim reaction. The cardinal immunologic defect in sarcoidosis seems, therefore, to be a depression of delayed type hypersensitivity which is readily demonstrated by skin tests using tuberculin, *Candida albicans*, or the chemical dinitrochlorobenzine (DNCB).

On the other hand, Israel and Sones (1967) found that in their patient material, the inability to develop and maintain tuberculin sensitivity which characterizes active sarcoidosis persists after the patients seemed to have made complete clinical and radiological recoveries from the disease. According to the same authors, the immunologic defect of patients with sarcoidosis, may be the result of systemic damage by the disease with the possibility that impaired ability to develop and maintain tuberculin sensitivity is a defect which antedates the development of sarcoidosis.

C. Role of Lymphocytes

In vitro culture of lymphocytes from sarcoidosis patients fails to show a normal blastic transformation in response to phytohemagglutinin (PHA).

SHARMA *et al.* (1970) correlated the *in vivo* dinitrochlorobenzine (DNCB) sensitization with *in vitro* lymphocyte transformation in 21 patients with histologically confirmed sarcoidosis, and an equal number of matched control subjects. Failure to sensitize with DNCB was noted in 71 % of sarcoidosis patients and 14 % of controls. Poor lymphocyte transformation occurred in 86 % of patients with sarcoidosis, and in only one of control subjects. The twin defects were a feature of 71 % of patients with sarcoidosis, indicating that *in vivo* cutaneous anergy reflects the *in vitro* cellular hyporeactivity.

LANGNER *et al.* (1969) studied the *in vitro* behavior of peripheral lymphocytes incubated with phytohemagglutinin. The transformation of lymphocytes was markedly inhibited in all cases of active sarcoidosis of the lung. The inhibition affected the earlier stages of transformation, as was shown by the markedly depressed percentage of mRNA, and then DNA synthesizing cells in culture. The inhibition was independent of the extent of the disease, but was correlated with its activity. During remission, the level of PHA stimulated transformation rose by a statistically significant margin.

It is interesting to note that lymphopenia often occurs in sarcoidosis. HOFFBRAND (1968) found that one-third of patients with sarcoidosis had blood lymphocyte counts less than 1,000/cu. mm. It was also noted that lymphocyte counts were related to tuberculin skin reactivity and that lack of reaction to tuberculin was associated with significantly lower levels of lymphocytes. HOFFBRAND found that peripheral blood lymphopenia of less than 1,000 per cu. mm was found in 20 of 61 patients with sarcoidosis compared with only one of 100 hospital control subjects. It was suggested that lymphocyte count in sarcoidosis provides a crude quantitative guide to the degree of impairment of delayed hypersensitivity. The level of circulating blood lymphocytes may also be of prognostic value as lymphopenia was found more often in the severer and more extensive forms of sarcoidosis.

The lymphopenia of sarcoidosis remains unexplained. It is possible, however, that this is due either to an *in vivo* defect of lymphocytes of patients with sarcoidosis which parallels the *in vitro* defect of lymphocytes in response to non-specific mitogens, or to a massive mobilization of lymphocytes as the blood-borne precursors of epithelioid cells.

VI. Hypercalcemia

Hypercalcemia and hypercalciuria have frequently been observed in patients with sarcoidosis and may on occasion lead to the development of nephrolithiasis, nephrocalcinosis and metastatic calcinosis in other parts of the body, such as the lungs (LATHAN *et al.*, 1968). BELL *et al.* (1964) studied the calcium, phosphorus and nitrogen balance in four patients with sarcoidosis and hypercalcruria following the administration of prednisone, vitamin D, and of both drugs. The effect of the same dosages of vitamin D was also examined in two normal subjects. In three patients studied without treatment, the fecal calcium level was low, the urinary calcium level high and serum antirachitic activity low or normal. In all four patients, fecal calcium levels could be decreased further without the abnormal increase in serum antirachitic activity following the administration of vitamin D. Vitamin D had no effect on either fecal calcium or calcium absorption in normal subjects. Prednisone therapy diminished both the spontaneous absorption of calcium and that produced with vitamin D. The results suggest that abnormal calcium metabolism in sarcoidosis is probably the result of an abnormally increased sensitivity to vitamin D rather than hypervitaminosis D per se.

More recently there has been interest in the finding of concomitant sarcoidosis and hyperparathyroidism (Winnacker et al., 1969 and Lief et al., 1969). Because sarcoidosis is often associated with hypercalcemia, an underlying parathyroid adenoma or primary hypoplasia may be easily overlooked. The association of hypercalcemia with significant hypophosphoremia should suggest hyperparathyroidism rather than sarcoidosis alone.

The current widespread use of corticosteroid in patients with sarcoidosis and the suppressive effects of these agents on sarcoid granuloma may explain the relative infrequency with which hypercalcemia is encountered in recent studies of patients with sarcoidosis (Goldstein et al., 1971).

On a morphologic basis, the presence of Schaumann bodies has not been correlated to the best of our knowledge with the level of hypercalcemia. The more recent observation of intramitochondrial dense and seemingly metallic bodies in epithelioid cells of sarcoidosis (Lunardelli, 1968) would suggest the possibility that such dense granules may contain calcium and may be a possible relation to the hypercalcemia of sarcoidosis.

VII. Conclusion: Sarcoidosis as a Reaction Pattern

Traditionally, the approach to the problem of sarcoidosis has been directed along two major lines: (a) One is aimed at finding a specific etiological agent. The following have been particularly investigated among others; atypical mycobacteria, lysed or altered mycobacteria, trace metals, pine pollen, etc. (b) An intrinsic defect in the lymphoreticular system, perhaps a genetic defect in lymphocytes partly translated into poor *in vitro* response to phytohemagglutinin and a defective delayed hypersensitivity to tuberculin.

It is obvious that the two approaches may be actually combined. In keloids, for example, the exaggerated collagenization is a genetic attribute but the stimulus is provided by injury no matter how trivial. Could a similar situation be present in sarcoidosis?

So far all attempts to incriminate one specific etiologic factor in sarcoidosis have either failed or did not succeed in gaining a wide credibility. On the other hand, there is no question, in our opinion, that we are dealing here with a condition in which an environmental factor is important. This is noticeable in that the distribution of the vast majority of sarcoid lesions suggest an environmental factor with certain predictable ports of entry. There is primarily an involvement of the upper respiratory tract, including cervical and mediastinal lymph nodes, and less frequently involvement of the lung parenchyma. Sarcoidosis of the skin, the uveal tract and of the parotid glands likewise suggest possibly an exposure to an exogenous factor. It is, of course, not entirely excluded that this exogenous factor may vary in quantity and type from case to case. Likewise, the disseminated forms of sarcoidosis often suggest a miliary hematogenous spread.

The presence of the peculiar pigment granules in the reticuloendothelial cells in lymph nodes harboring epithelioid granulomas in sarcoid patients deserves particular attention. The significance of these granules is not entirely clear. Their ultrastructural characteristics suggest that they represent residual bodies, probably resulting from autophagic digestion. The identification of nucleic acids in these pigment granules may signify the presence of a microorganism or nucleic acid derived from autophagic digestion of host nuclei or mitochondria.

The Kveim reaction presents a number of serious pitfalls which were not seriously considered a few years ago. It remains to determine precisely what a negative Kveim reaction is. There again we may be dealing with a quantitative degree of reaction rather than a qualitatively abnormal host reaction.

Finally, we are left with a concept of sarcoidosis which minimizes rather than disregards the importance of specific etiological factors. It is doubtful that we will ever discover one etiological factor accounting for the presently known forms of lesions now called sarcoid-type epithelioid granulomas. There are a number of "specific" granulomatous reactions associated with well-defined etiological agents. Other "specific" granulomas shall continue, in all probability, to be discovered. It is equally safe to predict that, in spite of future additions, there will remain a core of "sarcoid" noncaseating epithelioid granulomas of undetermined or uncertain etiology. To this group, one may add the epithelioid granulomas caused by endogenous products or by agents which are generally considered to be nonpathogenic or of doubtful pathogenicity, including atypical or lysed mycobacteria. In the final analysis, it is probably the host's reaction pattern rather than exogenous or endogenous offending agents that determines the epithelioid reactivity seen in patients with sarcoidosis.

References

AZAR, H. A.: Amyloidosis. Path. Ann. 3, 105–122 (1968).

AZAR, H. A., LUNARDELLI, C.: Collagen nature of asteroid bodies of giant cells in sarcoidosis. Amer. J. Path. 57, 81–92 (1969).

AZAR, H. A., MOSCOVIC, E. A., PHAM, T. D.: The fine structure of pigmented granules in RES cells of sarcoid lymph nodes. Fed. Proc. 29, 753 (1970) (Abstract).

BELL, N. H., GILL, J. R., BARTTER, F. C.: On the abnormal calcium absorption in sarcoidosis. Amer. J. Med. 36, 500–513 (1964).

BOWMAN, B. U.: Neutralization of mycobacteriophages by sera of patients with and without sarcoidosis. Proc. Soc. exp. Biol. (N.Y.) 129, 696–699 (1968).

BRINCKER, H.: Epithelioid-cell granulomas in Hodgkin's disease. Acta path. microbiol. scand., Section A 78, 19–32 (1970).

Buckley, C. E. III, Dorsey, F. C.: A comparison of serum immunoglobulin concentrations in sarcoidosis and tuberculosis. Ann. intern. Med. **72**, 37–42 (1970).

Buckley, M. P.: Historical aspects of sarcoidosis. Irish J. Med. Sci. **3**, 29–35 (1970).

Carter, C. J., Gross, M. A.: The selective staining of curious bodies in lymph nodes of patients as a means for diagnosis of sarcoid. Stain Technol. **44**, 1–4 (1969).

Celikoglu, S. I., Siltzbach, L.: A study of sarcoidosis and leprosy in Turkey employing the Kveim reaction. Dis. Chest **55**, 400–404 (1969).

Chapman, J. S., Speight, M.: Further studies of mycobacterial antibodies in the sera of sarcoidosis patients. Acta med. scand., Suppl. **425**, 61–66 (1964).

Cohn, Z. A., Fedorko, M. E., Hirsch, J. G., Morse, S. I., Siltzbach, L. E.: The distribution of Kveim activity in subcellular fractions from sarcoid lymph nodes. In: La Sarcoïdose. Rapports de la IVe Conference Internationale, p. 141–149. Paris: Masson & Cie 1967.

Cummings, M. M., Dunner, E., Williams, J. H., Jr.: Epidemiological and clinical observations in sarcoidosis. Ann. intern. Med. **50**, 879–890 (1959).

Daddi, G.: Immunologie de la sarcoïdose. Poumon **24**, 327–337 (1968).

Dumont, A., Sheldon, H.: Changes in the fine structure of macrophages in experimentally produced tuberculous granulomas in hamsters. Lab. Invest. **14**, 2034–2055 (1965).

Elias, P. M., Epstein, W. L.: Ultrastructural observations on experimentally induced foreign body and organized epithelioid cell granulomas in man. Amer. J. Path. **52**, 1207–1223 (1968).

Elling, P., Wanstrup, J.: Sarcoidosis. Immunohistological demonstration of immunoglobulin IgD in sarcoid lymph nodes. Acta path. microbiol. scand. **77**, 326–328 (1969).

Epstein, W. L., Krasnobrod, H.: The origin of epithelioid cells in experimental granulomas of man. Lab. Invest. **18**, 190–195 (1968).

Essner, E., Novikoff, A. B.: Human hepatocellular pigments and lysosomes. J. Ultrastruct. Res. **3**, 374–391 (1960).

Goldstein, R. A., Israel, H. L., Becker, K. L., Moore, C. F.: The infrequency of hypercalcemia in sarcoidosis. Amer. J. Med. **51**, 21–30 (1971).

Greenwood, R., Smellie, H., Barr, M., Cunliffe, A. C.: Circulating antibodies in sarcoidosis. Brit. med. J. **1958**I, 1388–1391.

Gusek, W.: Histologische und vergleichende elektronenmikroskopische Untersuchungsergebnisse zur Cytologie, Histogenese und Struktur des Tuberkulosen und tuberkuloiden Granuloms. Med. Welt **15**, 1–46 (1964).

Gusek, W.: Vergleichende Cytologie und Histogenese des Sarkoidosegranuloms. Arch. klin. exp. Derm. **227**, 24–53 (1966).

Gusek, W.: Formale Pathogenese der hyalinen Transformation des Sarkoidosegranuloms. Virchows Arch. Abt. A **345**, 264–275 (1968).

Hall, G., Sharma, O. P., Naish, P., Doe, W., James, D. G.: The epidemiology of sarcoidosis. Postgrad. med. J. **45**, 241–250 (1969).

Hardt, F., Wanstrup, J.: Sarcoidosis. An *in vitro* Kveim reaction based on the leucocyte migration test. Acta path. microbiol. scand. **76**, 493–494 (1969).

Harold, F. M.: Inorganic phosphate in biology: Structure, metabolism and function. Bact. Rev. **30**, 772–794 (1966).

Haroutunian, L., Fisher, A. M., Smith, E. W.: Tuberculosis and sarcoidosis. Bull. Johns Hopk. Hosp. **115**, 1–28 (1964).

Hirsch, J. G., Fedorko, M. E., Dwyer, C. M.: The ultrastructure of epithelioid and giant cells in positive Kveim test sites and sarcoid granulomata. In: La Sarcoïdose. Rapports de la IVe Conference Internationale, p. 59–70. Paris: Masson & Cie 1967.

Hirshaut, Y., Glade, P., Vieira, L. O. B. D., Ainbender, E., Dvorak, B., Siltzbach, L. E.: Sarcoidosis, another disease associated with serologic evidence for herpes-like virus infection. New Engl. J. Med. **283**, 502–506 (1970).

Hoffbrand, B. I.: Occurrence and significance of lymphopenia in sarcoidosis. Amer. Rev. resp. Dis. **98**, 107–110 (1968).

Israel, H. L., Goldstein, R. A.: Relation of Kveim-antigen reaction to lymphadenopathy. Study of sarcoidosis and other diseases. New Engl. J. Med. **284**, 345–349 (1971).

Israel, H. L., Sones, M.: The tuberculin reaction in patients recovered from sarcoidosis. In: La Sarcoïdose. Rapports de la IVe Conference Internationale, p. 295–298. Paris: Masson & Cie 1967.

James, D. G.: Historical aspects of sarcoidosis. Clio med. **3**, 265–271 (1968).

James, D. G.: Epidemiology and management of sarcoidosis. Practitioner **202**, 624–631 (1969).

James, D. G., Siltzbach, L. E., Sharma, O. P., Carstairs, L. S.: A tale of two cities. A comparison of sarcoidosis in London and New York: Arch. intern. Med. **123**, 187–191 (1969).

Kalifat, S. R., Bouteille, M., Delarue, J.: Étude ultrastructurale des altérations cellulaires et extracellulaires dans le granulome sarcoïdosique. In: La Sarcoïdose. Rapports de la IVe Conference Internationale, p. 71–88. Paris: Masson & Cie 1967.

Kalifat, S. R., Bouteille, M., Delarue, J.: Changes in connective tissue in sarcoid granuloma: hyalin, paraamyloid and fibrinoid. Electron microscopic study of 11 cases. Virchows Arch. Abt. B **3**, 348–358 (1969).

Kalkoff, K. W., Holtz, K. H.: Zur Mikromorphologie des intracytoplasmatischen Lipopigments (Ceroid) bei Sarkoidose und anderen Granulomen. Hautarzt **10**, 544–548 (1964).

Kang, K. S., Casida, L. E., Jr.: Large bodies of Mycoplasma and L-form organisms. J. Bact. **93**, 1137–1142 (1967).

Langner, A., Moskalewska, K., Proniewska, M.: Studies on the mechanism of lymphocyte transformation inhibition in sarcoidosis. Brit. J. Derm. **81**, 829–834 (1969).

Lathan, S. R., Block, R. A., McLean, R. L.: Sarcoidosis with "metastatic" calcification. Amer. J. Med. **44**, 1000–1004 (1968).

Lief, P. D., Bogartz, L. J., Koerner, S. K., Buchberg, A. S.: Sarcoidosis and primary hyperparathyroidism. Amer. J. Med. **47**, 825–830 (1969).

Löfgren, S., Ed.: Proceedings of the 3rd International Conference on Sarcoidosis. Acta med. scand., Suppl. **425**, 1–310 (1964).

Lordon, R. E., Young, R. L., Shapiro, S. S., Smith, R. E., Weg, J. G.: Sarcoidosis. II. A clinical evaluation of the alteration in delayed hypersensitivity. Amer. Rev. resp. Dis. **97**, 1009–1016 (1968).

Lunardelli, C.: Intramitochondrial bodies in epithelioid cells of sarcoidosis. Fed. Proc. **27**, 248 (1968) (Abstract).

Malkoff, D. B., Strehler, B. L.: The ultrastructure of isolated and *in situ* human cardiac age pigment. J. Cell Biol. **16**, 611–616 (1963).

Mankiewicz, E.: On the etiology of sarcoidosis. Canad. med. Ass. J. **88**, 593–595 (1963).

McDougal, S., Azar, H. A.: *In vivo* and *in vitro* uptake of tritiated proline by macrophages in foreign body granulomas. Arch. Path. In press (1971).

Mitchell, D. N., Cannon, P., Dyes, N. H., Hinson, K. F. W., Willoughby, J. M. T.: Further observations on Kveim test in Crohn's disease. Lancet **1970**II, 496–498.

Moscovic, E. A.: A histochemical and ultrastructural reappraisal of Hamazaki bodies in sarcoid lymphnodes; lipofuscin or a microbial L-phase. In preparation (1971).

Moscovic, E. A., Neptune, C. J. B.: Possible protozoal nature of pigment granules in RES cells of sarcoid lymphnodes. Fed. Proc. **28**, 549 (1969) (Abstract).

National Library of Medicine Literature Search. Mid 1963–Mid 1968. U.S. Department of Health, Education, and Welfare, Public Health Service, National Library of Medicine, Bethesda, Maryland. L. S. No. 17–66, 18–66, 19–66.

Okano, H., Khouri, F., Azar, H. A.: *In vitro* transformation of human lymphocytes into macrophages. Fed. Proc. **27**, 717 (1968) (Abstract).

Sharma, O. P., Fox, R. A., James, D. G.: Correlation of *in vivo* delayed-type hypersensitivity with *in vitro* lymphocyte transformation in sarcoidosis. Ann. intern. Med. **72**, 811 (1970) (Abstract).

Siltzbach, L. E.: An international Kveim test study 1960–1966. In: La Sarcoïdose. Rapports de la IVe Conference Internationale, p. 201–213. Paris: Masson & Cie 1967.

Siltzbach, L. E.: Sarcoidosis and mycobacteria. Amer. Rev. resp. Dis. **97**, 1–8 (1968).

Siltzbach, L. E.: Etiology of sarcoidosis. Practitioner **202**, 613–618 (1969).

Turiaf, J.: Anergie cutanée à la tuberculine et test de Kveim dans la sarcoïdose. Bull. Acad. Nat. Med. **152**, 91–99 (1968).

Turiaf, J., Battesti, J. P., Menault, M.: Anergie tuberculinique, test de Kveim et immunoglobulines seriques dans la sarcoidose. Poumon **24**, 625–645 (1968).

Turiaf, J., Chabot, J., Eds.: La Sarcoidose. Rapports de la IVe Conference Internationale, 782 pp. Paris: Masson & Cie 1967.

Vanek, J., Schwarz, J.: Demonstration of acid-fast rods in sarcoidosis. Amer. Rev. resp. Dis. **101**, 395–400 (1970).

Vogel, R. A.: Experimental pine pollen granuloma and serologic reactions with pine and mycobacterial antigens. In: La Sarcoïdose. Rapports de la IVe Conference Internationale, p. 499–503. Paris: Masson & Cie 1967.

Wanstrup, J.: Cellular and immunological reactions in sarcoid tissue; with a view to the morphogenesis of granuloma formation. Scand. J. Resp. Dis., Suppl. **65**, 243–250 (1968).

Wanstrup, J., Christensen, H. E.: Sarcoidosis. 1. Ultrastructural investigations on epithelioid cell granulomas. Acta path. microbiol. scand. **66**, 169–185 (1966).

Wanstrup, J., Elling, P.: Immunohistochemistry of sarcoidosis. Acta path. microbiol. scand. **73**, 37–48. **73**, 37–48 (1968).

Williams, W. J., Williams, D.: "Residual bodies" in sarcoid and sarcoid-like granulomas. J. clin. Path. **20**, 574–577 (1967).

Wilner, G., Abu Nassar, S., Siket, A., Azar, H. A.: Fluorescent staining for mycobacteria in sarcoid and tuberculous granulomas. Amer. J. clin. Path. **51**, 584–590 (1969).

Winnacker, J. L., Becker, K. L., Friedlander, M., Higgins, G. A., Moore, C. F.: Sarcoidosis and hyperparathyroidism. Amer. J. Med. **46**, 305–312 (1969).

Institute of Pathology, University of Hamburg
(Director: Prof. Dr. med. G. Seifert)

The Interepithelial Lymphocytes of the Intestinum. Morphological Observations and Immunologic Aspects of Intestinal Enteropathy

HERWART F. OTTO

With 14 Figures

Contents

I. Introduction

Distribution, position, cytomorphology, origin and fate of mononuclear lymphocytic cells within different epithelial layers have been the object of many investigations. Histotopographic and apparantly functional correlations have also been known for some time as the so-called migratory (mononuclear) cells (References: PATZELT, 1936). Previously much importance was attached to the occurrence of lymphocytic cells in the epithelial layer and many inter-

pretations have been suggested. The interest in such cell types is understandable
insofar as about 20% of the cellpopulation of the intestinal mucosa are not
epithelial cells; almost all of them are lymphocytes (Toner and Ferguson,
1971; Toner et al., 1971). Nakano (1931) claims that the values for interepithelial lymphocytes are 2.7% in the colon and 8.1% in the small intestine
(see also: Satake, 1924a, b; Jassinowsky, 1925). According to Darlington
and Rogers (1966) about 9% of the intestinal epithelial cells are lymphocytes
(see also: Toner, 1968).

The often speculative interpretation of the function of the lymphocytic
cells is due to the fact that the real functions of lymphocytes have only recently
been recognized. Since we known that the *small lymphocytes* are the essential
part of the immune reaction, many clinico-pathological and experimental
studies have been performed with the aim of providing clues to improved
understanding of function and morphology of interepithelial lymphocytes.

With reference to the immunologic importance of lymphocytes especially
in the gastrointestinal tract, I shall first describe the role of lymphocytes in
immunologic processes. Then I shall discuss the question of the lymphocytes
in the epithelial layer of the intestine with special reference to the literature
and our own results. The immunopathogenesis of different enteropathies will
be discussed in particular detail.

II. The Role of Lymphocytes in Immunologic Reactions

The lympho-reticular system of mammals represents an essential protection
against injurious effects of different foreign substances. Phagocytosis and
adaptive immunologic responses are important mechanism in this defensive
process. The phagocytosis is the older principle in phylogenesis (References:
Roos, 1970). Phylogenetic studies have shown that the development of specific
immunologic reaction to antigenic stimulation ("immunologic competence",
Medawar, 1960) corresponds to the development of lymphocytes (Good and
Papermaster, 1964; Good et al., 1966; Papermaster et al., 1964; Finstad
and Good, 1966; References: Cottier et al., 1969; 1970a, b, Hess, 1970).

On the basis of new investigations the so-called *small* lymphocytes definitely
appear to be a functionally heterogenous cell population (Trowell, 1958;
Bos, 1967; Yoffey, 1967). The majority of these cells seem to be involved in
immunobiological processes (References: Cottier et al., 1969). The small
lymphocytes can be divided into at least two different groups, the so-called
long-living and short-living cell populations. Special importance must be given
to the ability of long-living lymphocytes to enter the lymphatic system and/or
blood stream (Everett et al., 1964). This guarantees the migration into tissues
and the possibility of recirulation. Both these capacities, *permeation* and *recirculation*, are necessary for the overall presence of immunologic reactivity of
the lympho-reticular tissue in the body. One or more of the diverse immune
reactions may result from contact of immunocompetent lymphocytes with
antigenic (Nossal, 1969). Most of the immunoreactive cells are probably in

non-stimulated state. Antigenic material is necessary to promote stimulation and proliferation. Furthermore, it appears that the continous influence of the antigen is necessary not only for the initial transformation of small lymphocytes, but also for the subsequent division and differentiation cycles.

The antigenic stimulation of competent lymphocytes postulates a *surface-detection-mechanism*. One interpretation proposed suggested that competent lymphocytes possess antibody-like receptors which are able to react with the specific antigenic determinants (NOSSAL, 1968, 1969; NOSSAL *et al.*, 1962, 1963, 1965, 1968). Obviously concentration and presence are essential for the induction and maintenance of immunologic reactions. Probably these surface receptors are membrane-bound immunoglobulins or fragments of them (KLEIN *et al.*, 1968; LEVIN *et al.*, 1969; RAFF *et al.*, 1970). Recognition and stimulation necessitate changes in the metastable state of the membrane or the receptors (SMITHIES, 1968; FISCHER *et al.*, 1970).

Besides membrane-bound receptors the process of immunologic reactions requires interaction between immunoreactive cells; on the one hand between lymphocytes and lymphocytes and on the other between macrophages and lymphocytes. Experiments have shown that in the case of hapten-protein complexes for example, the protein carrier plays an essential part in the production of hapten-specific antibodies. MITCHISON (1967, 1969, 1970) observed that irradiated animals which were completely unable to produce an immune pattern showed an hapten-specific immune response to an injected hapten-protein complex only after they had received hapten-specific as well as carrier-specific memory lymphocytes from adequate immunized donor animals. The cells which act as carriers in this connection have a so-called nurse function. Probably the contact with hapten-specific cells depends upon antigen bridges. Obviously the nurse cells have the task of concentrating antigenic substances and have to transfer them in adequate form to antibody-producing cells.

I do not intend to discuss the interaction between macrophages and lymphocytes so will refer the reader to the publications of UNANUE and ASKONAS (1968, 1969), KÖLSCH and MITCHISON (1968), DRESSER (1968a, b) and ROOS (1970).

The cytotoxicity also seems to be essentially a membrane phenomenon. According to PERLMANN (1969), the intimate membrane contact between living lymphocytes and target cells is solely responsible for the cytotoxicity of the lymphocytes and for the destruction of the target cells (see also BERKE *et al.*, 1969). BRUNNER (1967, 1968), too, found in his model of allograft rejection that intimate cell-to-cell contact between sensitized lymphocytes and target cells is necessary before rejection can occur. Furthermore these intimate membrane contacts play a part not only in allogenic transplant rejections but also for autogenous cells in cases of autoimmunity (WATSON *et al.*, 1966; SHORTER *et al.*, 1968, 1969). LOEWENSTEIN *et al.* (1964, 1967, 1969) claims that the biochemical bonds between different cells are possible in so-called "nexus junctions" (WEINSTEIN, 1969). The intimate membrane contact apparently induces partial membrane "alterations" ("septate junctions"). Similar biochemical contact bonds between cytotoxic lymphocytes and target cells should be possible (see also Fischer *et al.*, 1970). In this sense the problem of interepithelial lymphocytes of the gastrointestinal tract seems to be a membrane problem.

III. History

Apparently *small round cells* in the basal portion of the epithelium were first describes as being initially young proliferating cells of the epithelium by Weber (1847). In later years these results were often corroborated. Eberth (1861) took these interepithelial migratory cells for mucous bodies which were thought to be produced in the epithelial cells and then expressed in a mature state. On the basis of later studies (1884), however, he decided they must be independent cells entering the epithelium from the subepithelial stroma. Eimer (1866) also maintained that the interepithelial migratory cells were endogenous in epithelial cells. Rindfleisch (1861), Koelliker (1867) and Lipsky (1867), also looked upon these cells as epithelial cells. Edinger (1877) seems to have been the first to interpret them as leukocytes. Watney (1877) saw a connection with fat absorption and emphasized that they do not lie within the epithelial cells but always between them. Stöhr (1883, 1889) described a certain metamorphosis of lymphocytic migratory cells as they moved through the epithelium (see also Wolf-Heidegger, 1939). He denied any connection between migratory cells and fat absorption.

For a long time there was controversy about the so-called transepithelial migration of the lymphocytes (lamina propria mucosae — lumen of the bowels). In 1864 Eberth wrote: "... that perhaps some of them migrated to the luminal surface of the mucous membrane and there became mucous body". v. Hessling (1866) as well thought that they were "lymphbodies" of the villous parenchyma which moved to the surface of the villi. In 1867 v. Arnstein observed the transepithelial migration process. Later the lymphocytic migration through the epithelium was confirmed by several studies (Stöhr, 1883, 1889; Oppel, 1897; Schaffer, 1927; Wolf-Heidegger, 1939). On the other hand v. Davidoff (1887), Muthmann (1913), Hellman (1934) and Stenquist (1934) rejected any such migration of lymphocytes.

Heidenhain (1888) studied the relation between interepithelial lymphocytes and different physiologic and pathologic conditions of the gut. Schaffer described mitoses of lymphocytes for the first time in 1891, whereas Weill (1920) emphatically rejected these.

First v. Arnstein (1867), then Beguin (1904), Guieysse-Pellissier (1911, 1912) and Goldner (1929) supposed that migratory cells might permeate into the intestinal epithelium. Besides a cytoplasmic mixture of both cell types the nucleus of the migratory cells had to be substituted for that of the epithelial cells (*caryoanabiosis*); a process which was correlated with the regeneration of the intestinal epithelium at least by Goldner (1929).

Comparative anatomic studies furthermore showed that apparently there were certain relations between quantity and cytomorphologic structure of the migratory cells on the one hand and digestive processes on the other. The fact that the intestinal epithelium contains many lymphocytic migratory cells during hibernation was observed by HEIDENHAIN (1888) in the Bat, by MONTI (1903) in the Marmot and by CORTI (1907) in the Hedgehog. CORTI (1907) claimed that only a very small cytoplasmic rim can be seen during hibernation, which becomes more conspicuous during digestion. Similar results were found by BEGUIN (1904) in the Paddock and in the Lizard.

Early investigations point to the fact that the number of lymphocytic migratory cells varies widely in different parts of the gut and that moreover it seems to depend on the digestive process. The interepithelial lymphocytes have repeatedly been linked with assimilative and absorptive processes. They were supposed to have the particular function of *transepithelial carriers* (gut lumen — chylus vessel) in fat absorption (EIMER, 1866, 1869, 1884; WATNEY, 1877; References: PATZELT, 1936). Partly these already are theories which were later called *trephocytic function* of the interepithelial lymphocytes on the suggestion of CARREL (1924) (HUMBLE *et al.*, 1956; KELSALL and CRABB, 1958, 1959; BRYANT, 1962; KOTANI *et al.*, 1967; SHIELDS *et al.*, 1969).

IV. The Interepithelial Lymphocytes of the Normal Intestinal Mucosa

A. The Lympho-Reticular Tissue of the Intestinal Wall

Interepithelial lymphocytes within the epithelial layer are located between (*inter*) the epithelial cells (WATNEY, 1877; MEADER and LANDERS, 1967; OTTO and MARTIN, 1971; OTTO and WALKE, 1972), within the gastrointestinal canal in preformed spaces, the so-called *intercellular space* (Fig. 1). In the intestinum these cells appear to be an integral part of the lympho-reticular system. Often these structures as a whole are considered as lympho-epithelial organ or tissue (MOLLIER, 1913; HARTMANN, 1914; JOLLY, 1919; WATZKA, 1932; FICHTELIUS, 1967, 1968; FICHTELIUS and JAROSLOW, 1969; FICHTELIUS *et al.*, 1969), functionally an independent tissue formation (DOERR, 1956). Especially the tunica propria mucosae is the seat of an ubiquitous lympho-reticular system. The reticular tissue of the stroma of the mucous membranes contains in lymphocytes and many other cell types the retiform spaces, including plasma-cytic, histiocytic, reticular and endothelial cells. Furthermore, defined aggregations of lympho-reticular structures are known, normally called lympho-noduli solitarii and Peyer's plaque (see also: ACKERMAN, 1962).

B. Appearance of Lymphocytes

Most of the interepithelial lymphocytes within the normal mucous membrane of the gut are *small lymphocytes* (Fig. 1) (WEILL, 1920; CORTI, 1922;

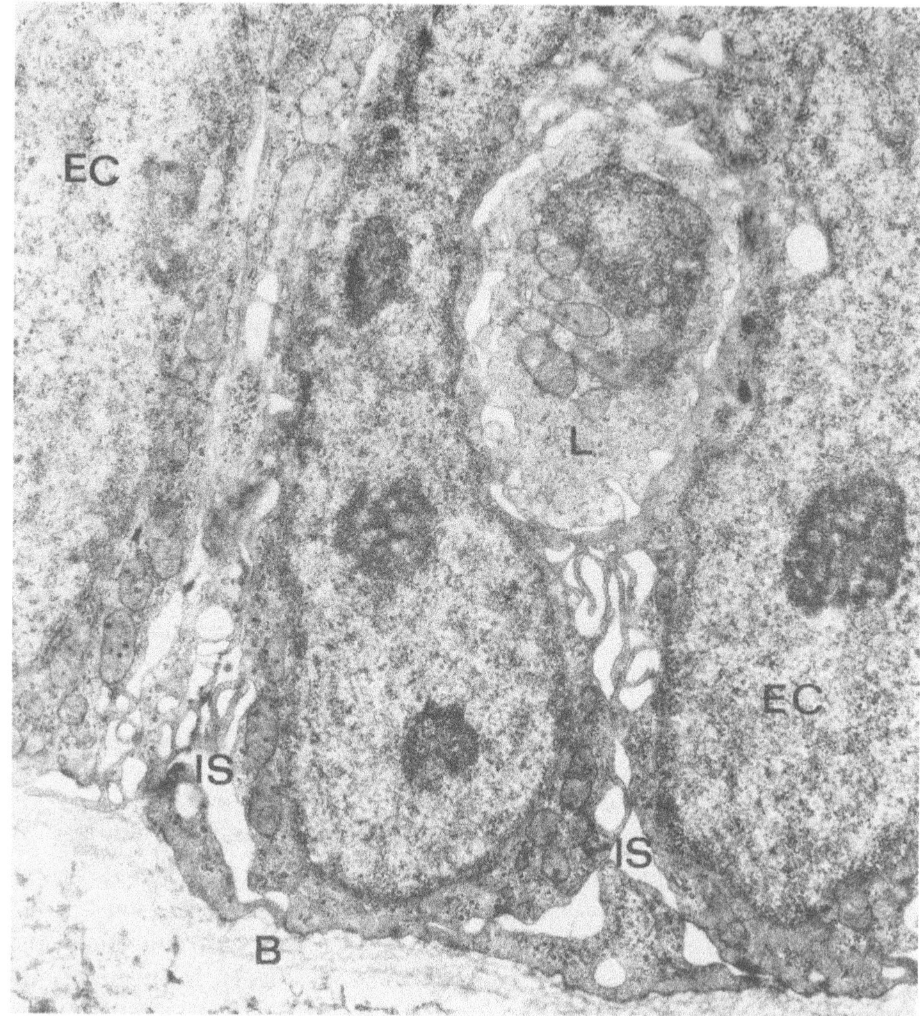

Fig. 1. Electron micrograph of the basal part of enterocytes from the normal human small intestine. Small interepithelial lymphocyte (*L*) between two epithelial cells (*EC*). Intercellular space (*IS*). Basement membrane (*B*). Magn. 12 500 ×

Jassinowsky, 1925; Schaffer, 1927; Törö, 1931; Stenquist, 1934; Wolf-Heidegger, 1939; Andrew, 1965; Andrew and Andrew, 1945; Andrew and Collings, 1946; Andrew and Sosa, 1947; Kelsall, 1946; Meader and Landers, 1967; Fichtelius *et al.*, 1969; Shields *et al.*, 1969; Otto and Martin, 1971; Otto and Walke, 1972; Walke, 1972).

In light microscopy these lymphocytes can be recognized as dark, chromatin-dense cells apparently devoid of cytoplasm (Fig. 2). Very occasionally a small cytoplasmic rim can be observed. As a rule the lymphocytes are surrounder by a broad clear ring visible on light micrographs. According to the electron microscope observation recorded by Meader and Landers (1967) this clear ring is composed of unstained, nongranular cytoplasm of the lymphocytes and of the surrounding intercellular space. Interepithelial lymphocytes are not, however confined to the intestine. Similar microscopy findings were obtained in other organs too: by BOHLE *et al.* (1970) and by VOGT *et al.* (1970) in normal human kidneys, in acute renal insufficiency as well as in peracute, chronic-proliferating and sclerosing glomerulonephritis and in kidney transplants; by

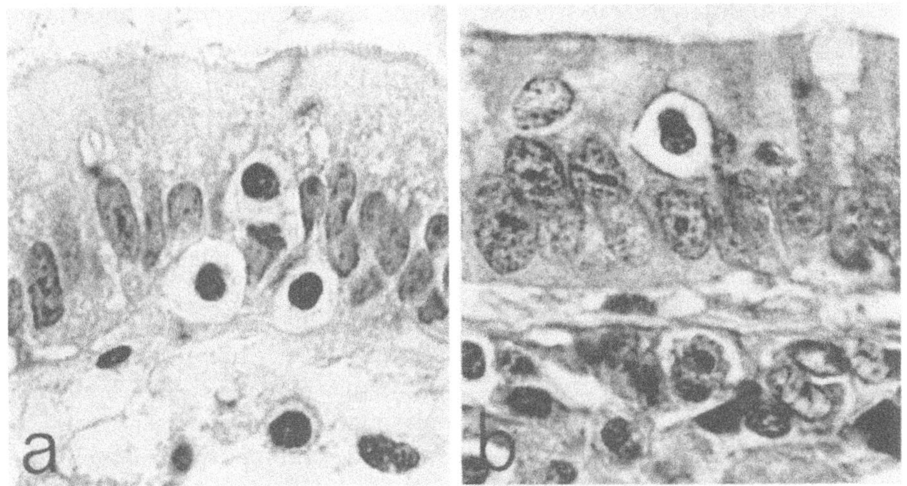

Fig. 2a and b. Light micrograph of intestinal villus from the normal jejunum. a Two interepithelial lymphocytes in the basal, and one interepithelial lymphocyte in the intermediate region. b One interepithelial lymphocyte in the apical position of the epithelium. The intercellular position of the lymphocytes is obvious from the presence of an "apparent clear ring". Hematoxylin and eosin. Magn. 1 370 ×

SHIELDS *et al.* (1969) both in the bronchial mucous membrane and in the endometrium. TOUJAS and GUELFI (1969) found these cells in the epidermis (see also: ANDREW, 1949; ANDREW and ANDREW, 1949; DARCY, 1952; BILLINGHAM and SPARROW, 1954; WAKSMAN, 1960; WIENER *et al.*, 1962, 1964), in the genitalia and also in the thyroid gland; HAYWARD *et al.* (1968) in the salivary gland and in the biliary tract.

Interepithelial lymphocytes with a pericellular light optically clear ring were observed too in the guts of different vertebrate animals (DARLINGTON and ROGERS, 1966; MEADER and LANDERS, 1967; FICHTELIUS *et al.*, 1969; OTTO, 1971 b).

PFEIFFER and WEIBEL (1969) identified similar cells in the antral-pyloric area of the ferret and called them *"antral clear cells"*. But although regarding their position and cytoarchitecture, these "antral clear cells" appear to be almost identical to the interepithelial lymphocytes, PFEIFFER and WEIBEL suspect an endocrine function. NEMETSCHEK-GANSLER and WAGNER (1969) take the so-called "small cell-infiltrates" for epithelial proliferations, which are said to be quite typical of regional enteritis (Crohn's disease) and coeliac sprue.

ANDREW and his co-workers (ANDREW, 1965; ANDREW and ANDREW, 1945; ANDREW and COLLINGS, 1946; ANDREW and SOSA, 1947) interpreted this clear ring as a degenerative change the lymphocytes (see also: TONER et al., 1971). Moreover ANDREW (1965) observed different morphologic appearances of the lymphocytes between villi and crypts (see: J. Nat. Cancer Inst. 35, 113, 1965; Fig. 1–3 and 12–16). According to these investigations there are also differences in the morphologic appearances of the lymphocytes in the stratum proprium mucosae and the epithelial layer. On the contrary both we (OTTO, 1971b; OTTO and MARTIN, 1971; OTTO and WALKE, 1972; WALKE, 1972) and MEADER and LANDERS (1967) did not observe such differentiations either in normal or diseased intestinal mucosa.

According to WIENER (1970), in thin sections the small lymphocytes are 5–6 μ in diameter; according to MORI and LENNERT (1969) 8 μ in diameter. In our own investigations we found apico-basal diameters of between 5.5 and 6.5 μ (OTTO and WALKE, 1972) and 7 and 8.5 μ (OTTO and MARTIN, 1971). By plain metric analysis on small lymphocytes of the ductus thoracicus of rat HEBEL and LIEBICH (1969) found the following mean values diameter of the cell: 4.2 μ, diameter of the nucleus: 3.3 μ, cytoplasmic plane: 5.3 μ², nucleolar plane: 0.75 μ². The mean nuclear-cytoplasmic ratio is represented by the index number 1.63. According to HEBEL and LIEBICH the cell volume is about 40 μ³, the cell surface of the "idealized cell globule" is 55 μ². The authors believe however, that the true values are a little higher.

The nuclei are usually round to ovoid. Occasionally small invaginations can be found. The nuclear chromatin is irregularly dispersed; some nuclei are euchromatic, some heterochromatic with dense chromatin condensations near the nuclear periphery. The nucleoli are often not visible. The small cytoplasmic rim contains few organelles: few mitochondria; a small amount of narrow Golgi channels and of rough-surfaced endoplasmatic reticulum; varying numbers of ribosomes. The numerous nonmembrane-associated ribosomes account for the cytoplasmatic basophilia of these cells (PALADE, 1958; SIEKEVITZ, 1959, 1961; FAWCETT, 1961). In interepithelial lymphocytes of normal intestinal mucosa we found centrioles, osmiophilic granules ("electron opaque lysosomal granules", WIENER, 1970; "small, dense homogeneous granules", TONER et al., 1971), multivesicular bodies, vesicles or vacuoles. MEADER and LANDERS (1967) published similar observations. The outer cell membrane is sometimes even and sometimes partly shows pseudopodal formations. The pseudopodal projections in particular show intimate membrane contact with epithelial cells, some of which may form the so-called "nexus-junctions" ("septate junctions") (LOEWENSTEIN, 1969; POLITOFF et al., 1969; WEINSTEIN, 1969; WEINSTEIN and SOMEDA, 1968), whose function in the normal mucous membrane is not yet fully understood.

In contrast, TONER and FERGUSON (1971) and TONER et al. (1971) found a greater morphologic variability of interepithelial lymphocytes. In regard to size, form and organelle equipment their results correspond to ours, found in enteric diseases.

C. Distribution and Position of Lymphocytes

According to our own investigations (OTTO and WALKE, 1972; WALKE, 1972) the number of interepithelial lymphocytes of the small intestine increases aborally, most of them being in the distal ileum and in the appendix. Earlier former investigations have already drawn attention to these quantitative differences within different parts of the intestine (References: PATZELT, 1936). In many cases the number of interepithelial lymphocytes was regarded as a function of migration. NAKANO (1931) graded the intensity of migration with the so-called *"migration coefficient"*:

$$\text{migration coefficient} = \frac{\text{number of interepithelial lymphocytes}}{\text{number of epithelial cells}}\%.$$

According to NAKANO (1931) this coefficient is 8.1 % for the small intestine, 4.2 % for the coecum, and 2.7 % for the colon. SATAKE (1924a, b) specified the number of migrating lymphocytes per day as 25–38 million for the small intestine, 1.5–7 million for the coecum and 4–6 million for the colon. Converted to numbers per 1 cm intestine the figures are as follows: 200000–290000; 300000–630000; 50000–76000. There seems to be a correlation between the number of emigrating lymphocytes on the one hand and point of time as well as food intake on the other. According to JASSINOWSKY (1925) the lymphocytic migration comes to 4700 lymphocytes per 7300 epithelial cells in the upper jejunum, to 7100 per 8000 epithelial cells in the ileum.

The means observed by MEADER and LANDERS (1967) were 15875 lymphocytes related to 2500 villi; by SHIELDS *et al.* (1969) 75 ± 6 small lymphocytes per 1000 mucous cells in malabsorption syndrome, pancreatic insufficiency, nontropical sprue and irritable bowel ("In patients whose jejunal mucosa was studied, such diagnoses were suspected, but the patients proved to be normal", SHIELDS *et al.*, 1969).

Table 1. Interepithelial lymphocytes per 1000 mucosal cells (from SHIELDS *et al.*, 1969)

	Interepithelial lymphocytes			
	Intact	Ballooning	Degenerate	Total
Range	22–42	7–12	26–40	64–87
Aritmetic mean	33.75	8.38	32.56	74.69
per cent	45	11	44	100
Standard deviation	5.67	1.63	3.60	6.01

These numbers correspond to ours in normal mucosa of the small intestine (see also: Fig. 5). Where cytoplasmic "ballooning" and degenerative alterations of the interepithelial lymphocytes were observed, mentioned also by ANDREW and co-workers, MEADER and LANDERS (1967) concluded that they might be fixation artefacts in light microscopy. This "clear ring" was observed by electron microscopy to be composed of the unstained and nongranular cytoplasm of the lymphocyte and the surrounding intercellular space. MEADER and LANDERS (1967) explain the presence of "clear ring" or "vacuoles"

(ANDREW *et al.*, 1945, 1946, 1947, 1965) around the lymphocytes on the basis of an *inter*cellular position. TROWELL's (1958) observations of this phenomenon in the intestinal epithelium of the rat, cat, dog and frog led him to support the claims of ANDREW (1945, 1965) and ANDREW *et al.* (1946, 1947).

The values of interepithelial lymphocytes were a little higher in comparative experimental studies on several animal species (see also: table 2 and 3). According to DARLINGTON and ROGERS (1966) 9 % of the cells in the epithelial layer of the small intestine of mice are interepithelial lymphocytes, more than 95 % of which are located below the level of the nucleus. Moreover, in auto-radiographic investigations with ^{3}H-thymidine and ^{35}S-sulphate by DAR-LINGTON and ROGERS (1966), the interepithelial lymphocytes turned out to be different from the epithelial cells. These results disproved the hypothesis that the lymphocytes were merely pycnotic epithelial cells.

Table 2. Distribution and number of intercellular lymphocytes within the intestinal epithelium of animals (from MEADER and LANDERS, 1967)

Animals	Total number of lymphocytes counted for 2 500 villi	Below level of nucleus		Above level of nucleus	
		No.	%	No.	%
Mice	19 150	18 925	98.8	229	1.2
Rats	18 600	18 191	97.8	409	2.2
Hamsters	16 950	16 323	96.3	627	3.7
Total	54 700	53 435	97.6	1 256	2.4

Table 3. Number of intercellular lymphocytes in epithelium of the villi in young and old C 57 BL mice (20 oil-immersion fields per animal) (from ANDREW, 1965)

Lymphocytes	Young animals	Old animals
Total number in epithelial layer	251.2 ± 14.43	112.50 ± 5.77
Number in process of degeneration	1.60 ± 0.40	1.00 ± 0.30
Percent of total in process of degeneration	0.63	0.89

Most of the interepithelial lymphocytes are located below the level of the epithelial cell nuclei, close to the basement membrane (MEADER and LANDERS, 1967) (see also: Table 4 and 7). Approximately 97.6 % of the total 54 700 lymphocytes considered for animals were distributed below the level of the epithelial cell nuclei, with 98.7 % of a total of 15 875 lymphocytes assuming this same distribution in the intestinal epithelium of man (MEADER and LANDERS, 1967). The results obtained by ANDREW (1965) are listed in Table 4.

Table 4. Position of intercellular lymphocytes in epithelium of the villi in young and old C 57 BL mice (20 oil-immersion fields per animal) (from ANDREW, 1965)

Position of lymphocytes in epithelium	Young animals	Old animals
Basal	207.30 ± 12.47	71.80 ± 5.60
Intermediate	30.25 ± 2.89	33.80 ± 2.75
Apical	12.30 ± 1.68	2.80 ± 0.56

Our examinations of human biopsy specimen of normal upper small intestine (mainly upper jejunum) revealed 63.412 ± 17.302 interepithelial lymphocytes per 1 000 epithelial cells, 67.13 % of which were located in the basal region, 24.29 % at or near the level of the epithelial cell nuclei, and 8.5 % in supranuclear (apical) position (see also: Table 7; OTTO and WALKE, 1972; WALKE, 1972). But we never observed interepithelial lymphocytes at the level of the terminal web, the microvilli or in the lumen of the bowels.

The predominantly basal position of interepithelial lymphocytes can be found in the epithelial layer of other organs too. In investigations on several renal diseases (BOHLE et al., 1970; VOGT et al., 1970), the values for lymphocytes in infranuclear (basal) position ranged from 78–94 %, in intermediate position from 5–20 % and in supranuclear (apical) position from 1 to 2 %.

D. Eosinophils, Mast Cells and Globule Leucocytes

Oucasional *interepithelial eosinophils* stand in the same general relationship to the epithelial cells as the lymphocyte just described. They have the typical features of the eosinophil, including the compound inclusions with a characteristic crystalline bar (Fig. 3 and 4). Apparently these cells are more frequently found in animals than in man. Their cytoplasm contains scanty granular endoplasmatic reticulum and quite plentiful smooth-surfaced vesicles. Their

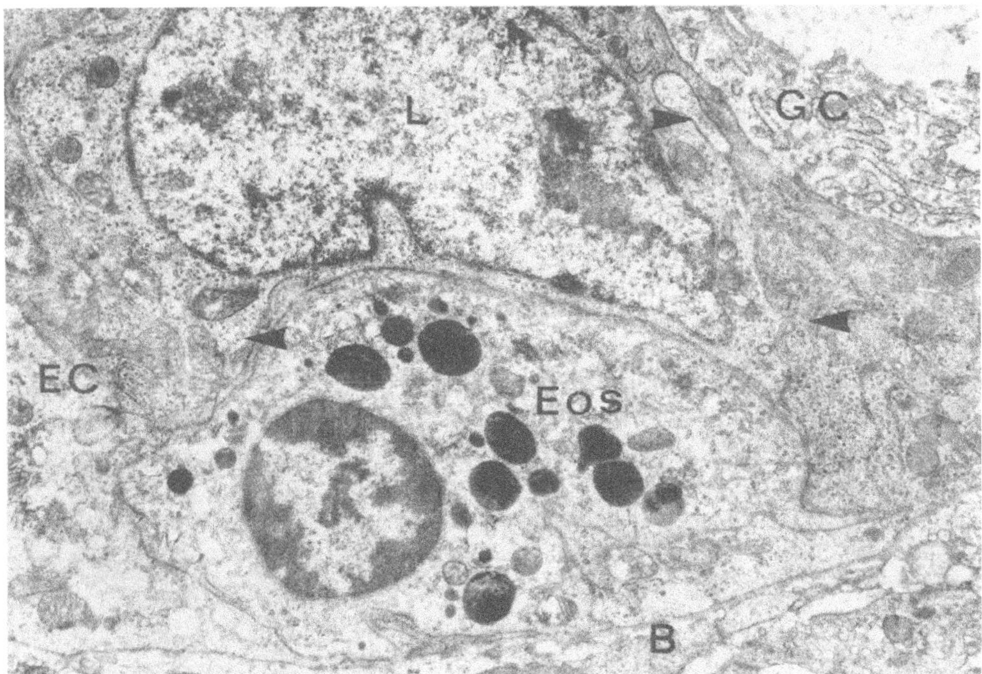

Fig. 3. Electron micrograph of interepithelial eosinophil (*Eos*) and lymphocyte (*L*). Human large bowel from patient with ulcerative colitis. The eosinophil and the lymphocyte have an irregular amoeboid outline, with pseudopodia extending between epithelial cells (*EC*) and goblet cells (*GC*). Basement membrane (*B*). Magn. 13 000 ×

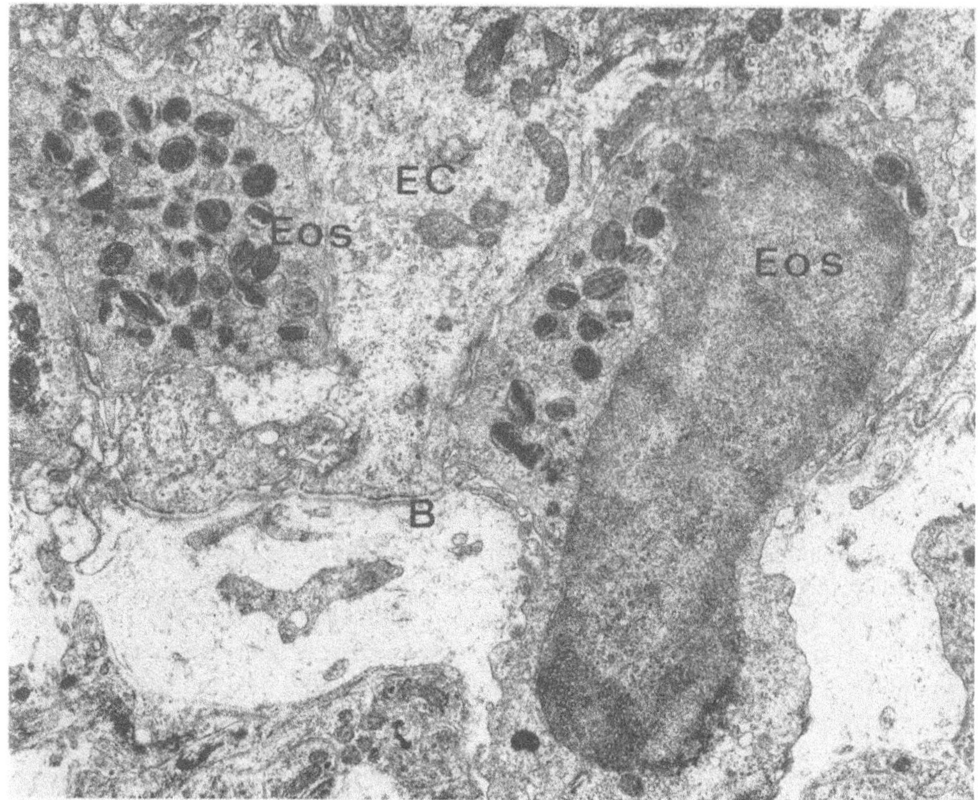

Fig. 4. Electron micrograph of a interepithelial and a migrating eosinophils (*Eos*). Human large bowel from patient with ulcerative colitis. Epithelial cells (*EC*). Basement membrane (*B*). Magn. 15000 ×

nuclear and cytoplasmic features are in general comparable to those of the eosinophils of the lamina propria.

Interepithelial mast cells in man (DOBBINS *et al.*, 1969) are rounded in outline with small surface projections folded flat by pressure from adjacent cells. They have the typical granules of the mast cell (STOECKENIUS, 1956; LOW and FREEMAN, 1958; BLOOM, 1965; ASTALDI *et al.*, 1966; WEINSTOCK and ALBRIGHT, 1967; SCHAUER and GERSTER, 1970). They are membrane-limited, pleomorphic inclusions containing amorphous and granular areas, empty areas and variable numbers of tubular laminated structures with a complex scroll-like pattern on transverse section (THIERY, 1963; WEINSTOCK and ALBRIGHT, 1967; BRINKMAN, 1968; DOBBINS *et al.*, 1969). Similar inclusions are described elsewhere as characteristic of human mast cells (THIERY, 1963; FEDORKO and HIRSCH, 1965; WEINSTOCK and ALBRIGHT, 1967; BRINKMAN, 1968; DOBBINS *et al.*, 1969). These cells are basally positioned and have been observed by the present authors in human stomach and intestine.

Globule leucocytes have been recorded by histologists over many years in various situations (KIRKMAN, 1950; KENT, 1952, 1966; KELLAS, 1961; TONER,

1965, 1968; Silva, 1967; Carr, 1967; Carr and Whur, 1968; Takeuchi *et al.*, 1969). This is an easily recognized interepithelial cell. The globule leucocyte is most commonly found in the digestive tract, but is also seen in the epithelium of the gall bladder, trachea, urinary bladder and genital tract of various species. The nature and function of the globule leucocyte are not known. The globule leucocyte resembles the interepithelial lymphocyte in that it appears to be essentially migratory or transient in type. In this case, there is more evidence that the cells reach the lumen of the gut. It has been alleged that globule leucocytes may originate in lymphocytes, plasma cells or mast cells. While there are certain structural similarities between globule leucocytes and lymphocytes, it is more difficult to relate globule leucocytes to plasma cells. Fine structure alone is, however, an unsatisfactory basis for the establishment of cell relationships. Recent work has suggested that the globule leucocyte may be a modified form of the atypical subepithelial mast cell (Murray *et al.*, 1968), a view supported by both ultrastructural and cytochemical data.

V. The Lympho-Epithelial Relationship of Intestinal Enteropathy, Especially of Idiopathic Steatorrhoea, Ulcerative Proctocolitis and Crohn's Disease

A. Introduction

Detailed morphologic analyses about lympho-epithelial relations in enteric diseases are comparatively rare. Earlier investigations have emphasized physiologic aspects of the digestive process (see also III. History): Schäfer (1884) considers general assimilative and absorptive processes. Stöhr (1891/92) in particular claimed connections with the removal and excretion of dissimilating body material. de Waele (1899), Zietzschmann (1905), Hellman (1934) and Stenquist (1934) emphatically expressed the opinion that the lymphocytic cells lying in the epithelial layer have a protective function against bacterial invasion of the gut. Additional support seems to be lent to this by the investigations of Glimstedt (1933) who used animals reared in sterile conditions. According to Hellman (1934), Glimstedt (1933) and Stenquist (1934) the occurrence of lymphocytic cells in the enteric epithelial layer is the result of the normal intestinal flora. Despite these conclusions that bacteria induce migration of interepithelial lymphocytes, morphologic studies on quantity and cytoarchitecture of lymphocytes in enteric diseases have been neglected for quite some time. Only since the research of Fichtelius and his co-workers (Fichtelius, 1967, 1968; Fichtelius and Jaroslow, 1969; Fichtelius *et al.*, 1969) have lympho-epithelial relations been considered as possible pathogenic immune reactions too. These studies originated in an attempt to find an equivalent of the Bursa Fabricii in birds. The function of the Bursa Fabricii-dependent lymphatic tissue can be seen in the production of immunoglobulins and antibodies. Although all vertebrates are known to have this Bursa-dependent lymphocytic function this organ was only found in birds.

Therefore it seems reasonable to postulate an ubiquitous lympho-epithelial equivalent. FICHTELIUS and co-workers studied the occurrence of lymphocytes in the intestinal mucous membranes of vertebrates with different phylogenetic age ("theliolymphocytes"; FICHTELIUS *et al.*, 1969). They found the so-called theliolymphocytes in close proximity to the basement membrane of the epithelial layer. SHIELDS *et al.* (1969) studied lympho-epithelial relations in the jejunal mucosa in malabsorption syndrome, pancreatic insufficiency, non-tropical sprue and irritable bowel (see also Table 1). MARKS *et al.* (1966, 1968), later LAGUENS *et al.* (1971) pointed out the large number of interepithelial lymphocytes in dermatitis herpetiformis. In the region of the oral mucous membranes repeatedly intensive lymphomonocytic infiltrates were described in the Behcet's syndrome (LEHNER, 1969; SAITO *et al.*, 1971).

B. Distribution and Number of Lymphocytes

Our own analysis (OTTO and MARTIN, 1971; OTTO and WALKE, 1972; WALKE, 1972) of lympho-epithelial relations in different enteric diseases is shown in Table 5.

Table 5. Review of investigated intestine specimen (from OTTO and WALKE, 1972). Control biopsies in parenthesis

Diagnoses	Number of cases
1. Normal small intestine	87
2. Non-specific enteropathy	76
3. Whipple's disease	7 (13)
4. Idiopathic steatorrhoea	34 (21)
5. Ulcerative proctits	23 (34)
6. Ulcerative colitis	54
7. Crohn's disease	11
8. Normal rectal mucosa/ non-specific proctitis	13
9. Cancer of colon	8

The quantitative results of our studies are listed in Table 6.

Idiopathic steatorrhoea ("coeliac sprue", RUBIN *et al.*, 1962), Crohn's disease and ulcerative colitis or proctocolitis are characterized by their high values of interepithelial lymphocytes (see also Fig. 5). The values are related to the acute, untreated stage of idiopathic steatorrhoea and to the first manifestation or to acute exacerbations of ulcerative proctocolitis (see also WALKE, 1972). In contrast to our results SHIELDS *et al.* (1969) observed the same values both in malabsorption syndrome and nontropical sprue and in normal mucosa and other inflammatory conditions of the gut. We never found primary ballooning or degenerative changes of interepithelial lymphocytes in enteropathy. Only in regions of ulcerations or abscess formation in the crypts in Crohn's disease

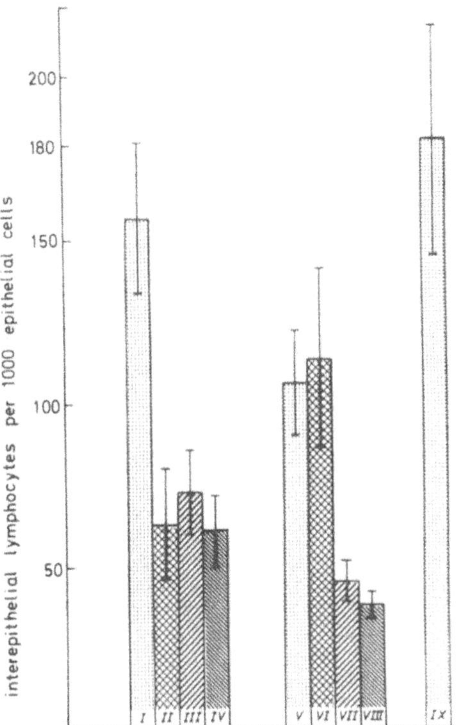

Fig. 5. Number and standard deviation of interepithelial lymphocytes of the normal intestinal mucosa and intestinal enteropathies in human. *I* idiopathic steatorrhoea; *II* normal small intestine; *III* non-specific enteropathy; *IV* Whipple's disease; *V* ulcerative proctitis; *VI* ulcerative colitis; *VII* normal rectal mucosa and non-specific proctitis; *VIII* cancer of colon; *IX* Crohn's disease

and ulcerative colitis did we observe degenerative alterations of interepithelial lymphocytes attributable to localized mucous lesions.

Calculation of the statistic significances of different correlations (for example ulcerative proctitis—normal rectal mucosa, Crohn's disease—normal small intestine) with Student's t-test yielded values significant at the 99% level (probability of error = 1%) (OTTO and WALKE, 1972).

C. Position of Lymphocytes

Although in general the position of interepithelial lymphocytes in the gut epithelium in enteropathies corresponds to that in normal mucous membranes there is an increase in the number of these cells (Table 7).

Apart from a prominent accumulation in the basal region there are only a few interepithelial lymphocytes at or above the levels of the nuclei. Quite often the lymphocytes resemble pearls in a necklace. The position of the lymphocytes is *inter*cellular (see also MEADER and LANDERS, 1967).

Table 6. Interepithelial lymphocytes per 1 000 epithelial cells in enteropathies and normal intestinal mucosa. Mean ($\bar{x}$), standard deviation (S_x), standard error of the mean ($s_{\bar{x}}$), possible limit of error (pe_x) and possible limit of error of the mean ($pe_{\bar{x}}$). Number of cases (n). (from OTTO and WALKE, 1972)

Diagnoses	n	$\bar{x}$	s_x	$s_{\bar{x}}$	pe_x	$pe_{\bar{x}}$
1. Normal small intestine	87	63.412	17.302	1.855	11.671	1.215
2. Non-specific enteropathy	76	73.125	13.320	1.528	8.984	1.031
3. Whipple's disease	7	61.234	11.052	4.102	7.454	2.766
4. Idiopathic steatorrhoea	34	157.278	27.031	4.636	18.232	2.576
5. Ulcerative proctitis	23	106.609	16.309	3.401	11.000	2.294
6. Ulcerative colitis	54	113.315	28.062	3.819	18.928	2.516
7. Crohn's disease	11	180.909	35.896	10.823	24.212	1.300
8. Normal rectal mucosa/ non-specific proctitis	13	45.154	5.900	1.636	3.979	1.104
9. Cancer of colon	8	38.625	3.852	1.362	2.598	0.919

Table 7. Interepithelial lymphocytes per 1 000 epithelial cells in enteropathies and normal mucous membranes. Mean ($\bar{x}$) with standard detion (s_x) and position in the epithelial layer (from OTTO and WALKE, 1972)

Diagnoses	Total number ($\bar{x}$; s_x)	Position in epithelium		
		Basal %	Intermediate %	Apical %
1. Normal small intestine	63.412 ± 17.302	67.13	24.29	8.58
2. Non-specific enteropathy	73.125 ± 13.320	59.89	28.89	11.14
3. Whipple's disease	61.234 ± 11.052	73.03	25.31	1.66
4. Idiopathic steatorrhoea	157.278 ± 27.031	67.91	28.92	3.17
5. Ulcerative proctitis	106.609 ± 16.309	70.10	25.03	4.87
6. Ulcerative colitis	113.315 ± 28.062	66.97	26.92	6.11
7. Crohn's disease	180.909 ± 35.869	63.83	29.74	6.43
8. Normal rectal mucosa/ non-specific proctitis	45.154 ± 5.900	71.39	24.87	3.74
9. Cancer of colon	38.625 ± 3.852	62.80	32.36	4.84

D. The Cytological Ultrastructure of Lymphocytes

In idiopathic steatorrhoea, ulcerative proctocolitis and Crohn's disease at least some of the interepithelial lymphocytes increase distinctly in size (Fig. 6). The diameter increases from between 8.1 and 10.2 µ to 10.0 and 12.0 µ (OTTO and MARTIN, 1971; OTTO and WALKE, 1972). The results inferred from illustrations in work by TONER and FERGUSON (1971) and TONER et al. (1971). Unfortunately these authors do not mention whether the mucous membrane was normal or diseased.

The interepithelial lymphocytes in idiopathic steatorrhoea, ulcerative proctocolitis and Crohn's disease have about the same diameter as activated lymphocytes or immunoblasts (WIENER, 1970). In the literature there are various synonyms for them: transitional cells (FAGRAEUS, 1948), large lympho-

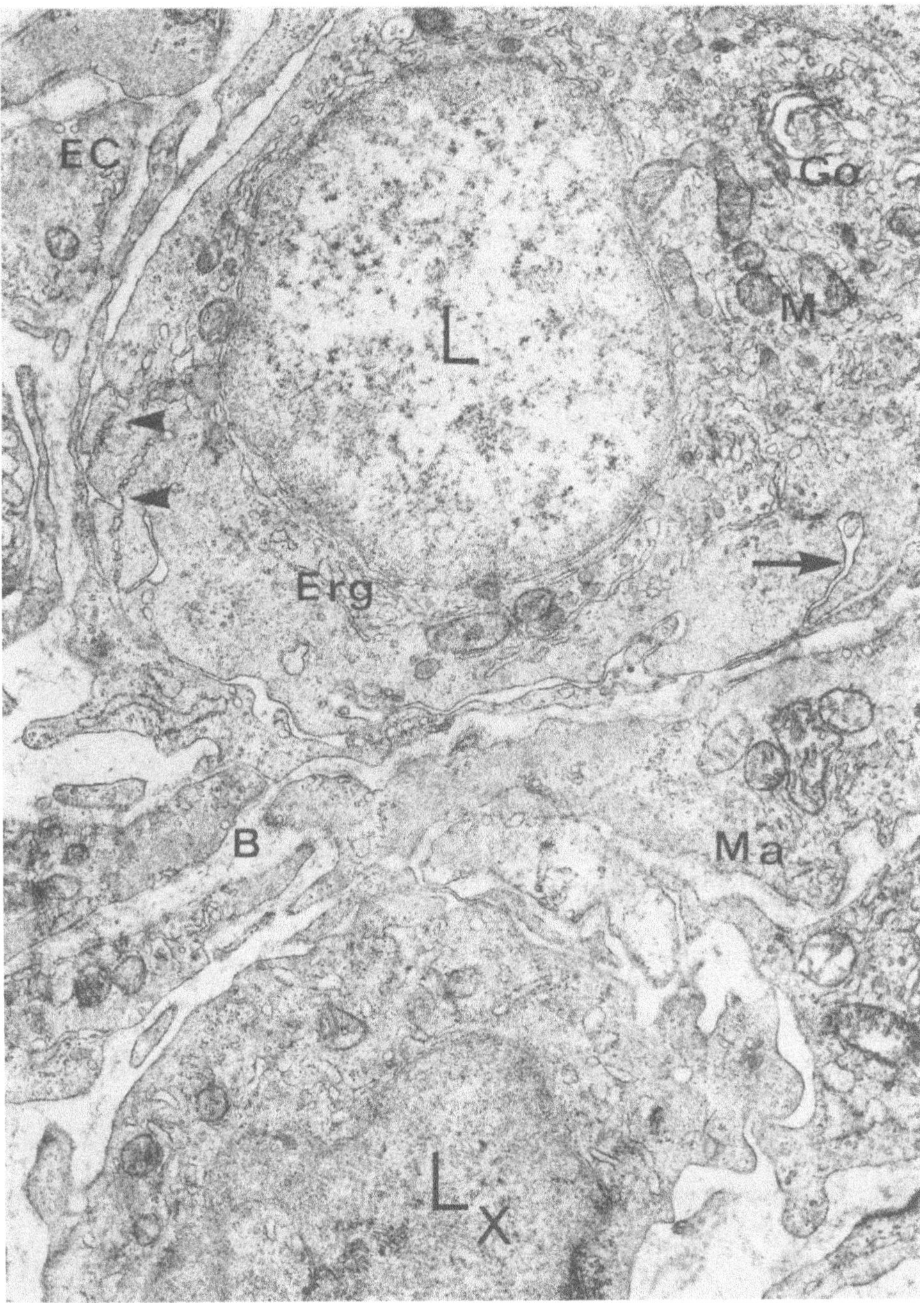

Fig. 6. Electron micrograph of an activated (=immunoblast) interepithelial lymphocyte (*L*). This activated lymphocyte has a round, euchromatic nucleus, a prominent Golgi complex (*Go*), several mitochondria (*M*) and large numbers of free ribosomes and polysomes. Several cisternae of rough surfaced endoplasmic reticulum (*Erg*) and an extensive system of pinocytotic vacuoles (short arrows) are present in the cytoplasm. It has an irregular amoeboid outline, with pseudopods often penetrating deeply into the cytoplasm (long arrow) of the epithelial cells (*EC*). Basement membrane (*B*). Macrophage (*Ma*) and activated lymphocyte (*L$_x$*) in the lamina propria. Magn. 12500 ×

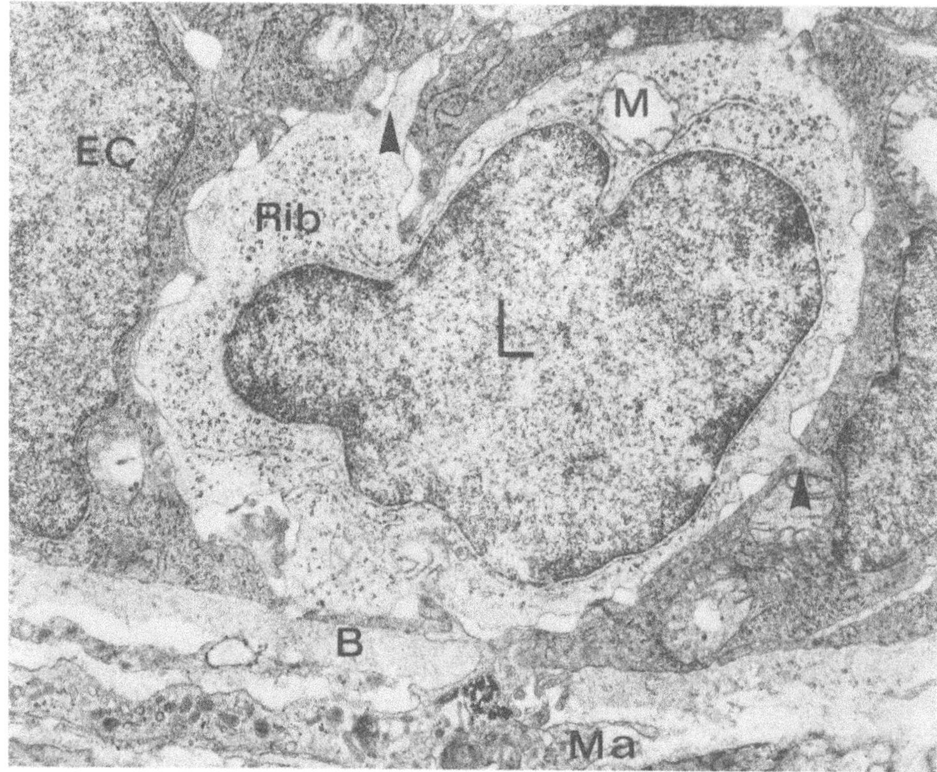

Fig. 7. Electron micrograph of an activated interepithelial lymphocyte (L) from a patient with ulcerative proctocolitis. The caryoplasma is leptochromatic with an irregular invaginated membrane. Large numbers of free ribosomes (Rib) and polysomes, single mitochondria (M) and surfaced endoplasmic reticulum are present in cytoplasm. The lymphocyte has an amoeboid outline with pseudopods extending between adjacent cells (arrows). Epithelial cells (EC). Basement membrane (B). Macrophage in (Ma) the lamina propria. Magn. 13 515 (from Otto and Walke, 1972)

cytes (Trowell, 1958; Nossal and Mäkelä, 1962), activated reticular cells (Marshall and White, 1950), large pyroninophilic cells (Gowans et al., 1962), hemocytoblasts (Fagraeus, 1960) and blasts (Nossal and Mitchell, 1963; Dameshek, 1963). Even in regard to their ultrastructure the large interepithelial lymphocytes are quite similar to immunoblasts.

Nucleus

Generally the nucleic have differently deep invaginations (Fig. 7, 9). The caryoplasm is usually leptochromatic. Quite seldom there are heterochromatic nuclei with coarse and denser chromatin condensations at the margin. Furthermore, granular deposits of ribosomal size can be seen in the caryoplasm. In contrast to our results, nuclear bodies were a rather frequent observation in studies by Andrew (1965), Meader and Landers (1967), Toner and Ferguson (1971) and Toner et al. (1971).

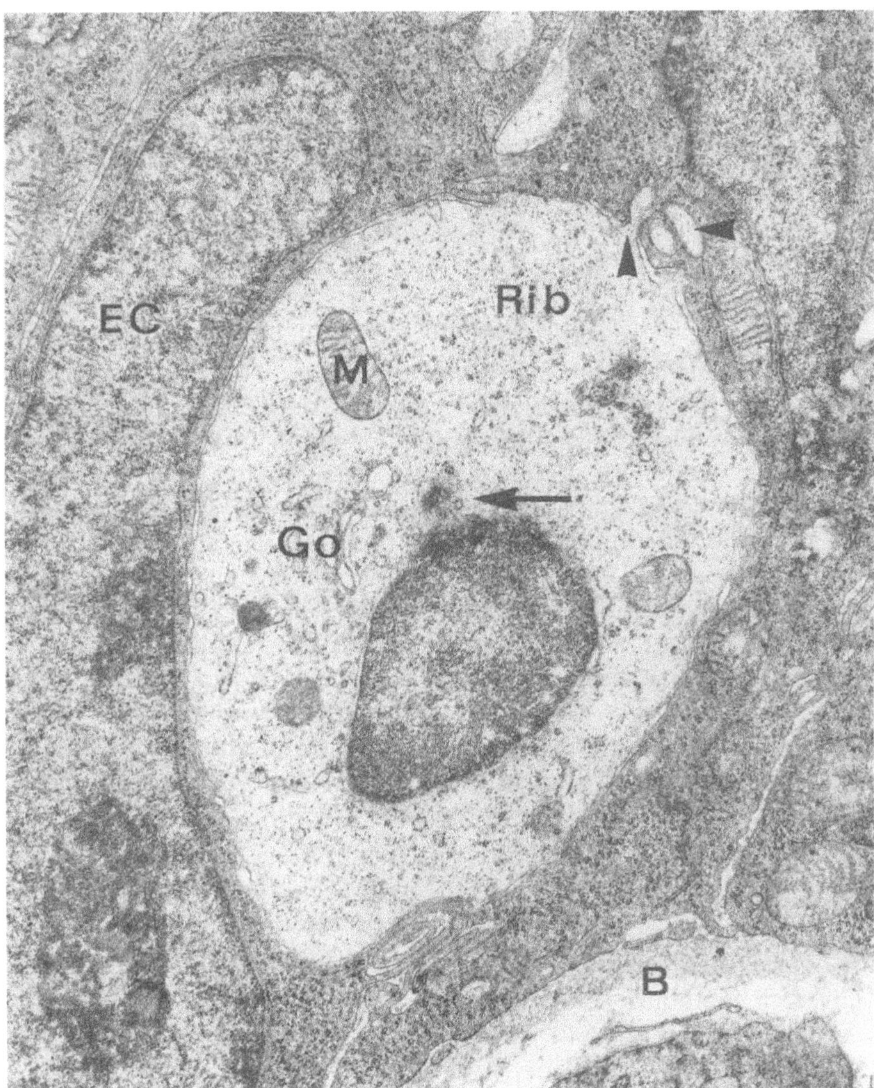

Fig. 8. Electron micrograph of an activated interepithelial lymphocyte from a patient with idiopathic steatorrhoea. Large numbers of free ribosomes (*Rib*) and polysomes, a prominent Golgi complex (*Go*), single mitochondria (*M*) and osmiophilic granules are present in the cytoplasm. Satellite-like outpouching of the caryoplasma (long arrow) and nuclear pores can be seen. The membrane contact between lymphocyte and epithelial cells is intimate, with single pseudopods (short arrows). Epithelial cells (*EC*). Basement membrane (*B*). Magn. 15700 × (from OTTO and WALKE, 1972)

The nuclear envelope consists of two membranes which are divided by a perinuclear cysterna, sometimes forming saccular structures. On the outer surface numerous ribosomes are deposited in rows or spirals. Along the nuclear surface the perinuclear cysterna shows so-called nuclear pores, the position of which is indicated by small light areas within the otherwise homogeneously

7*

dispersed chromatin. The quite constant finding of such light areas opposite to the pores repeatedly served as an indirect proof of metabolic passages (WATSON, 1959; AFZELIUS, 1963; STEVENS and SWIFT, 1966; KESSEL, 1966). Besides the invaginations satellite-like outpouching of the caryoplasm is seen very frequently (Fig. 8). At the border of the caryoplasmatic satellites and of the surrounding cytoplasmic ground substance small vesicles can often be found.

Ribosomes and Polysomes

The cytoplasm contains many free ribosomes, frequently associated to form polyribosomes (polysomes). The number of the ribosomes and polysomes is much higher than the number of (small) interepithelial lymphocytes of normal mucous membrane. In infectious hepatitis SIRTORI (1967) and ASTALDI *et al.* (1969) observed the transformation of lymphocytes to pyroninophilic cells migrating in the intercellular spaces of the jejunal epithelial layer. The pyroninophilia depends on the increase in ribosomes and polysomes, seen by light microscopy, as is proved by electron microscopy (see also PALADE, 1958; SIEKEVITZ, 1959, 1961; FAWCETT, 1961). Surprisingly, a small cytoplasmic rim often lacks these organelles. According to MEADER and LANDERS (1967) this nongranular cytoplasmic rim partly causes the so-called "clear ring" of ANDREW (1965). Small vesicles partly communicating with the cell membrane seem to be multiplied in this homogeneous cytoplasmic zone. The ribosomal and polyribosomal density seems to decrease overall.

Endoplasmatic Reticulum

A small amount of lamelles of rough-surfaced endoplasmatic reticulum is usually seen in tubular formations (Fig. 6–9). Butt TONER and FERGUSON (1971) and TONER *et al.* (1971) observed also vesicular form of endoplasmatic reticulum also.

Golgi Complex and Centrioles

The Golgi complex, disposed near the nucleus is quite prominent in contrast to the small lymphocytes of the normal intestine mucosa (Fig. 6) (see also ANDREW, 1965; MEADER and LANDERS, 1967; TONER and FERGUSON, 1971; TONER *et al.*, 1971). It comprises a varying number of parallel membranes with differently-sized vacuoles at the poles. At both sides many small vesicles collect in a somewhat concave collection around the centrally-located lamelles. The Golgi complex is often related to the centrioles, which consist of typical "triplet structures", partly also of pericentriolar bodies, the so-called satellites. One end of the centriole seems to be closed; the interior is partly granulated and electron density is high throughout.

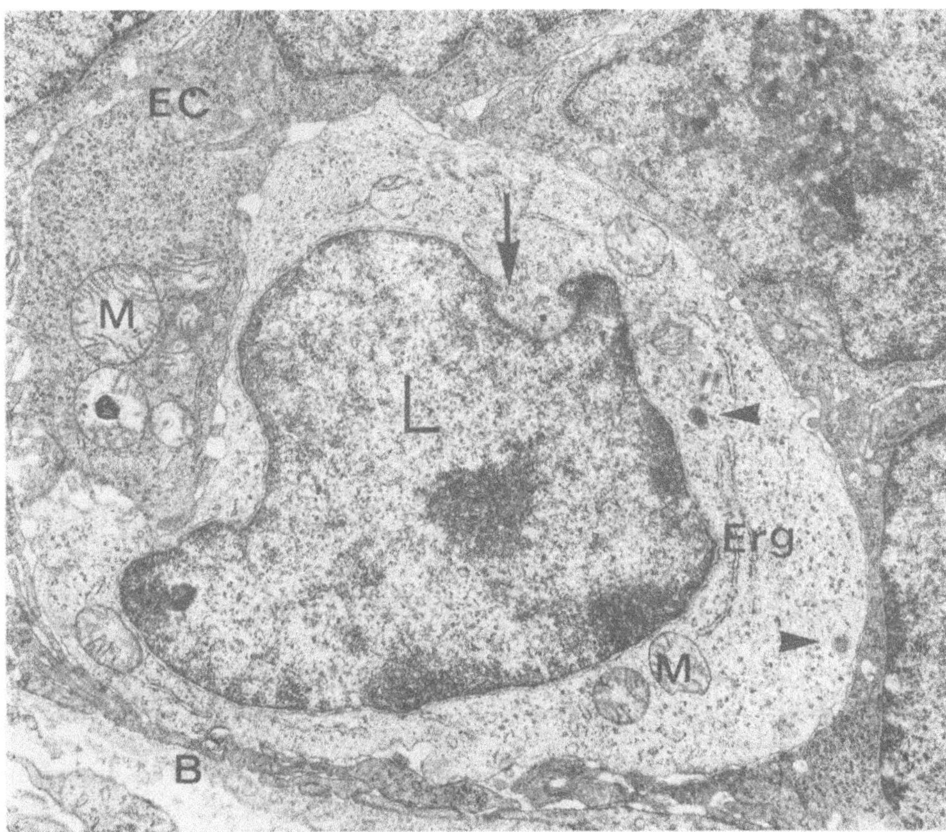

Fig. 9. Electron micrograph of an activated interepithelial lymphocyte (L) from a patient with ulcerative proctitis. This lymphocyte has a large, heterochromatic nucleus with invaginations, satellite-like outpouching of the caryoplasm and several nuclear pores (long arrow). Rough surfaced endoplasmic reticulum (Erg), mitochondria (M), free ribosomes and osmiophilic granules (short arrows) are present in cytoplasm. Epithelial cells (EC). Basement membrane (B). Magn. 13000 × (from OTTO and WALKE, 1972)

Osmiophilic Granules and Multivesicular Bodies

Small, mainly opaque osmiophilic granules are regularly distributed throughout the cytoplasm (Fig. 8, 9), the number varying from lymphocyte to lymphocyte. Some of these granules lie isolated, others form clusters (see TONER and FERGUSON, 1971; TONER et al., 1971). The solitary granules are usually bounded by a single membrane. They are thought to be "lipid droplets" (ANDREW, 1965). MEADER and LANDERS (1967) speak of relatively uniform, membrane-bound electron dense bodies. The last-mentioned authors, as well as TONER and FERGUSON (1971) and TONER et al. (1971), claim on the basis of their morphologic appearance that they are lysosomes.

According to TONER and FERGUSON (1971) and TONER et al. (1971) multivesicular bodies are a frequent finding.

Mitochondria

The mitochondria were few to moderate in number and dispersed at random in the cytoplasm (Fig. 6–9).

Cell Membrane

The lymphocytic cell-membrane builds up the contact surface with the adjacent epithelial cells. The relationship between these two membranes is of special interest (see also TONER *et al.*, 1971). Lymphocytic and epithelial cell membranes are in close approximation. Nearly the whole surface of the lymphocyte is involved in this membrane contact (Fig. 7–10). The intercellular space, in contrast to normal intestinal mucosa, is almost completely, filled up by lymphocytes. While ANDREW and JERSILD (1964) and ANDREW (1965) observed desmosomal junctions between lymphocytes and epithelial cells (J. Nat. Cancer Inst. *35*, 1965; Fig. 10 and 11), TONER and FERGUSON (1971) and TONER (*et al.* 1971) emphatically deny any specialized adhesion zones such as desmosomes or other close junctions between these cells. Nor did our own studies too ever reveal such desmosomes. More interesting, however, are interepithelial "nexus junctions" (WEINSTEIN and SOMEDA, 1968; WEINSTEIN, 1969) ("septate junctions", LOEWENSTEIN and KANNO, 1964; LOEWENSTEIN, 1967, 1969; POLITOFF *et al.*, 1969) in regard to the possible function of interepithelial lymphocytes. FARQUAHR and PALADE (1963) have described three morphologically distinct types of junctional complex of the intestinal epithelium: tight junction (zonula occludens), intermediate junction (zonula adhaerens) and the desmosome (macula adhaerens). Apparently such junctional complexes between interepithelial lymphocytes and adjacent epithelial cells do exist, nor is it likely that there are fusions of membranes. Nevertheless the term "caryoanabiosis" (v. ARNSTEIN, 1867; BEGUIN, 1094; GUIEYSSE-PELLISSIER, 1911, 1912; GOLDNER, 1929) necessarily implies membrane fusion as much as cell fusion. Also the occurrence of an *intra*cellular position of lymphocytes observed by TROWELL (1958) apparently postulates dehiscences of membranes. The same can be said of the *intra*epithelial position of lymphocytes repeatedly claimed by ANDREW (1965).

In our own material we encountered areas of contact surfaces which allowed no exact identification or distinction of two cell membranes even in electron microscope pictures of grade- and serial sections. But as we never observed lymphocytes in an intracellular position, as did MEADER and LANDERS (1967), we could not expect so-called membrane flows or membrane- or cell-fusions. It may be possible that there are structural alterations at molecular level in both cell membranes which form a so-called communication attachment without the cells being fused. But these nexus junctions apparently show an altered osmiophilia. Such membrane bridges permit a permeation of ions and even larger molecules from one cell to the other; according to LOEWENSTEIN (1969) the molecular size can reach molecular weights of about 1 000. The proof of such linkages has been supplied by microelectrodes (LOEWENSTEIN *et al.*, 1964, 1967, 1969). In non-linked cells the electric resistance is high and be-

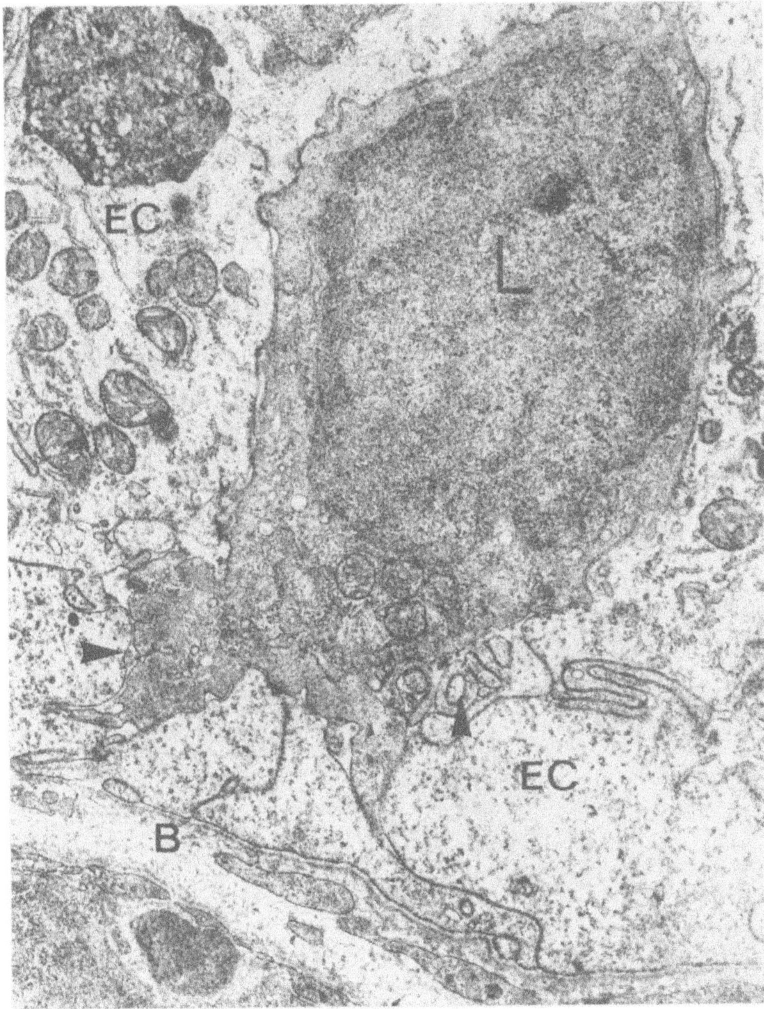

Fig. 10. Electron micrograph of an activated interepithelial lymphocyte (*L*) from a patient with Crohn's disease. The lymphocyte in this micrograph has marked irregularily of outlines, with several irregular pseudopods (arrows) pushing between and indenting the epithelial cells (*EC*). Basement membrane (*B*). Magn. 9000 ×

comes low in those with the cell linkages described above. Supposing that the interepithelial lymphocytes are immunocompetent cells, the trigger-mechanism of an immune response could possibly depend on similar membrane linkages. According to SMITHIES (1968) the cell membranes and receptor structures are in a metastable state of rest. The attachment of the hapten to the cell membrane alters this state, by giving energy to the membrane-receptor system, the morphologic equivalent of which could possibly be a distorsion of membranes. The lymphocyte could be activated by distorsion energy in excess of the minimum requirement. In regard to monovalent haptens the so-called "receptor removal model" is under discussion (SMITHIES, 1968).

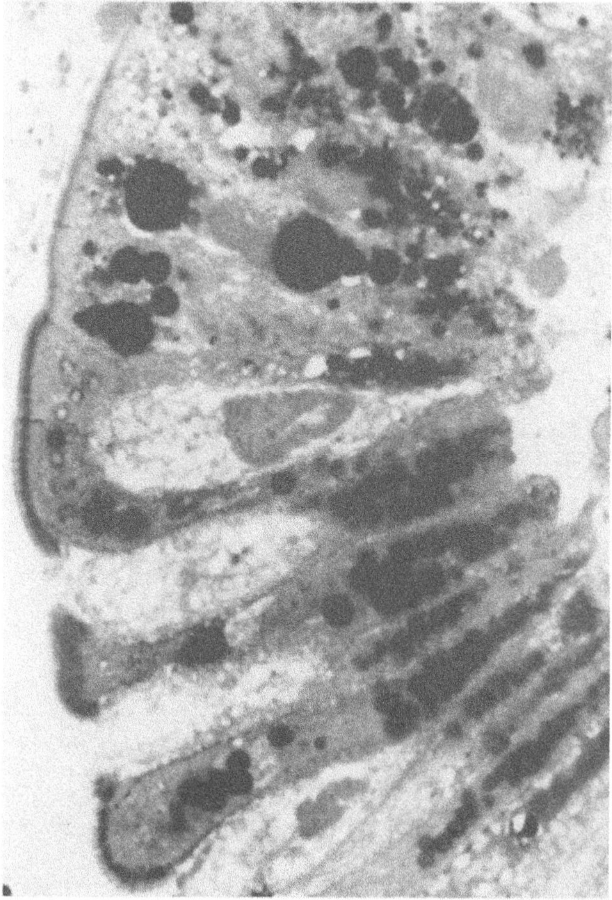

Fig. 11. Light micrograph of a epon-embedded semi-thin slide of rectal biopsy obtained from a patient with untreated ulcerative proctitis. Portions of goblet and columnar cells can be seen. The columnar cells contain inclusions ranging from dense (secretory) granules (aggregates of immunoglobulins?). The apical part of columnar cells showing several microvilli. Magn. 1 500 ×

Although the exact function of the interepithelial lymphocytes remains unknown (see also V. F.: Fate and function of lymphocytes) the intimate membrane contacts, which are only seen to this extent in idiopathic steatorrhoea, ulcerative proctocolitis and Crohn's disease, allow the conclusion of an immunocompetent and possibly of a cytotoxic function of these cells.

As well as linear membrane contacts there are also wound membrane contacts caused by pseudopodal outpouching of the cells (Fig. 6, 10) (see also ANDREW, 1965; MEADER and LANDERS, 1967; TONER and FERGUSON, 1971; TONER et al., 1971). TONER et al. (1971) observed extraordinarily variable partly irregular ameboid contures with many pseudopods of various lengths, which make deep indentations in the cytoplasm of the adjacent epithelial cells. But obviously there also are interdigitations of epithelial outpouching into the cytoplasm of lymphocytes (Fig. 7, 10).

E. Origin of Lymphocytes

The origin of interepithelial lymphocytes is not yet known. Former concepts claiming that lymphocytic cells are differentiations of intestinal epithelial cells are only of historial value (EBERTH, 1861; EIMER, 1866; RINDFLEISCH, 1861; KOELLIKER, 1867; LIPSKY, 1867). Nor can the hypothesis of HERMANS (1967) that lymphocytic cells, as well as absorbing differentiated intestinal epithelial cells, have their origin in primitive pluripotent intestinal epithelial cells, be maintained. Many observations lead to the conclusion that the lymphocytes migrate from the stratum proprium mucosae into the epithelial layer: for example studies by MEADER and LANDERS (1967), TONER *et al.* (1971) as well as our own show a rupture of the basement membrane and of collagen fibrils at the site of migration. The ameboid movements of interepithelial lymphocytes (TONER *et al.*, 1971) and the close correlation between the intensity of the cellular inflammation and the number of interepithelial lymphocytes (WALKE, 1972) also favour this conclusion. Last but not least the usually basal position of lymphocytes supports the above concept that the nucleus of the lymphocytes precedes the cytoplasm while moving from the lamina propria mucosae into the epithelium. LEWIS (1931) claimed that it has to be an active migration. TONER and FERGUSON (1971) and TONER *et al.* (1971) were also able to show that the nucleus with a small pseudopodal cytoplasmic rim apparently always breaks through the basement membrane while the remaining cytoplasm streams behind in an ameboid fashion.

v. ARNSTEIN (1867) and WOLF-HEIDEGGER (1939) have already mentioned the active (ameboid) lymphocytic migration into the intestinal epithelial layer. KELSALL (1946) speaks of ameboid movement in relation to migration of lymphocytes in the intestinal epithelium of the hamster. PALAY and KARLIN (1959), in an electron microscopic study of fat absorption, found lymphocytes and eosinophils in the process of entering the epithelium from the lamina propria apparently between the cells. WATZKA (1932) saw the migration as a passive process, according to which the lymphocytes flow with the lymph current into the epithelial layer. ANDREW and ANDREW (1945) also supposed this concept of passive movements.

Autoradiographic studies by HALL and SMITH (1970) indicated, however, that after antigenic stimulation many lymphocytes and immunoblasts enter the intestinal mucous membrane from non-intestinal lympho-reticular tissues.

F. Fate and Function of Lymphocytes

TONER *et al.* (1971) write (p. 178): "The origin and functions of these intra-epithelial lymphocytes are obscure. Various possibilities have been raised in the past; they might be in the course of migration from the lamina propria to the lumen; they might degenerate within the epithelium (ANDREW and ANDREW, 1945; ANDREW and SOSA, 1947; ANDREW, 1965; SHIELDS *et al.*, 1969); they might even transform into epithelial cells. There is inadequate evidence available to resolve the problem."

The problem of the fate of the interepithelial lymphocytes is a problem of their function.

In a recent article on lymphocytes in the intestinal epithelium, Andrew and Andrew (1945) review a number of theories: that the lymphocytes carry a thymic hormone; that they are the source of enzymes for lipids, or nucleins; that they are a factor in resistance either to bacterial toxins, to microorganisms, or to cancer.

De Waele (1899), Zietzschmann (1905), Hellman (1934) and Stenquist (1934) assume a general protective function of the interepithelial lymphocytes against the physiologic bacterial flora of the gut. Additional support for this concept is seen in studies by Glimstedt (1933), who besides other alterations saw a lack of germfree animals. There is much evidence that interepithelial lymphocytes together with specialized epithelial cells, for example the Paneth cells (Otto, 1971a, Otto and Weitz, 1972; Weitz, 1972) represent a dynamic regulative for the maintenance of the bacterial homeostasis of the gut. The active symbiosis between epithelial cells and interepithelial lymphocytes postulated by Jolly (1919), Braus (1924) and previously by Mollier (1913) remains hypothetic, though in connection with immunologic reactions (in different enteropathies) it is again increasing in importance.

According to Toner et al. (1971) the interepithelial lymphocytes of the small intestine generally have a bigger diameter than those in the circulating pool and the lymphoid tissues. Our own investigations, however, indicate that this is true only of inflamed intestinal mucosa, especially in ulcerative colitis, Crohn's disease and idiopathic steatorrhoea. In these diseases the interepithelial lymphocytes are comparable with the lymphocytes after Phythaemagglutinin-stimulation (Tanaka et al., 1963; Parker et al., 1965). Fichtelius (1967, 1968) concludes that the diffuse lympho-epithelial organ of the gut is a functional and morphologic analogue to the Bursa Fabricii in birds. According to Tonner et al. (1971) this concept implies that the contact between the two cell types (epithelial cells—lymphocytes) is very important in the development of immunologic competence of the immature lymphocytes. By way of comparison the lymphocytic cells of the normal intestinal mucosa could represent the morphologic equivalent of a "low-grade immune response" to the many food- and bacterial antigens of the gut. The distinct membrane contacts between normal epithelial cells and small lymphocytes could possibly be the "septate junctions" and "nexus junctions" postulated by Weinstein and Someda (1968; see also Weinstein, 1969) and Loewenstein (1969) which allow a flow of antigens from the absorbing epithelial cells to the lymphocytes. In this sense the active biologic symbiosis between the two cell types supposed by Mollier (1913), Jolly (1919) and Braus (1924) would undergo an amazing relevant interpretation.

According to Fichtelius (1967, 1968), Fichtelius et al. (1969), Ginsberg (1971) and other authors the gastrointestinal tract is a lympho-epithelial organ, comparable to the thymus and the Bursa Fabricii. The immunologically competent cells of the intestinal tract produce many immunolgobulins: IgG,

IgA, IgM, IgD and IgE (SLANEY, 1968; HOUSLEY *et al.*, 1969; WATSON, 1969a, b; HALL and SMITH, 1970; BOURNE *et al.*, 1970; STILLMAN and ZAMCHECK, 1970; ROGERS, 1970; GINSBERG, 1971) (see also Fig. 12). IgA is formed in plasma cells of submucosa and enters secretory epithelial cells of the gut (SOUTH *et al.*, 1968; TOMASI, 1968). In the epithelial cell 2 or 3 molecules of IgA combine to form a beta-globulin, the socalled transport piece (= secretory piece). This complex of IgA and transport piece is called secretory IgA and is secreted onto the luminal surface of the mucosa (Fig. 12). The exact role of transport piece is not known.

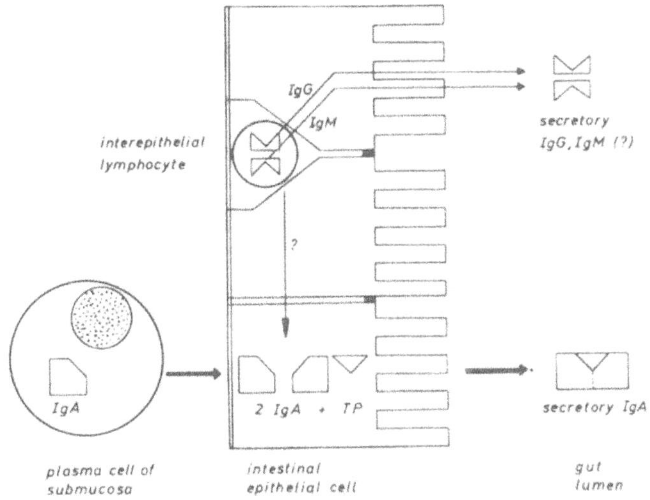

Fig. 12. Probable sequence of events in synthesis and secretion of secretory IgA of of (theoretical) IgG and IgM. *TP* Transport piece (see also Fig. 11)

According to HALL and SMITH (1970) specific antibodies are synthesized by large basophil cells (immunoblasts) located in the lamina propria of the gut. These cells are rich in ribosomes and polysomes and poor in endoplasmatic reticulum. Their cytoarchitecture often resembles that of activated interepithelial lymphocytes. In fluorescence-serologic studies with Anti-IgA, Anti-IgG and Anti-IgM serum biopsies of the small intestine in nontropical sprue revealed a clearly raised number of cells containing immunoglobulin (SØLTOFT, 1970). Especially the number of IgM- and IgG-producing cells was increased.

According to SOUTH *et al.* (1967), in salivary glands the synthesis of specific antibodies is regulated in three different ways: by local stimulation, systemically or by a combination of both (see also HURLIMANN, 1971). Possibly there could be a similar regulation in the gastrointestinal tract. Comprehensive reviews on the immunological system of all the mucous membranes are given by TOMASI and BIENENSTOCK (1968), HEREMANS (1968) and TOMASI (1970). GELZAYD *et al.* (1968) also reported the presence of immunoglobulins in the apical part of epithelial cells in human rectal glands and referred to a unique type of local immunoglobulin system, though they were uncertain of its biological significance. SCHOFIELD (1970) described columnar cells with secretory granules in the large intestine of the macaque (Cynamolgus irus) (see also Fig. 11). SCHOFIELD (1970) believes the protein nature of these granules to be proved and assumes aggregations of immunoglobulins within them (see also Fig. 12). For the production of idiopathic steatorrhoea, ulcerative proctocolitis and Crohn's disease immune and autoimmune mechanisms have been discussed. Possibly these correspond to an increased or atypical synthesis and secretion of immunoglobulins, besides the so-called cell mediated immunity (References: GINSBERG, 1971).

Idiopathic steatorrhoea (coeliac sprue; gluten enteropathy; non-tropical sprue): The concept of an immunologic or allergic reaction to gluten is based on the following observations:

1. Antibodies to gluten have been demonstrated in patients with idiopathic steatorrhoea (KIVEL et al., 1964; ALARCON-SEGOVIA et al., 1964; KATZ et al., 1968; HERSKOVIC et al., 1968; see also MIETENS, 1967a, b; MIETENS et al., 1971; HOBBS et al., 1969; IMMONEN et al., 1966; VISAKORPI and IMMONEN, 1967; ASQUITH et al., 1969);

2. Immunoglobulin and lymphocyte abnormalities are common in this disease (ASQUITH et al., 1969; BLECHER et al., 1969; BROWN et al., 1969; HOBBS et al., 1969);

3. There is a high incidence of lymphoproliferative disorders and neoplasm in idiopathic steatorrhoea (HARRIS et al., 1967);

4. Antibodies to gliadin have been identified within epithelial cells fluorescence microscopy. (RUBIN et al., 1965; RUBIN, 1971;

5. Steroids have a favourable effect on this disease (LEPORE, 1958; WALL et al., 1970).

Ulcerative proctocolitis: There are essentially two phenomena indicative of immunologic or autoimmunologic reactions in the development of ulcerative colitis:

1. Circulating anti-colon-antibodies (CORNELIS, 1958; BROBERGER and PERLMANN, 1959; BREGMAN and KIRSNER, 1960; ASHERON and BROBERGER, 1961; THAYER et al., 1969; LAGERCRANTZ et al., 1968; PERLMANN et al., 1967);

2. Lymphocytes with cytotoxic effects on allogenic colon tissue (WATSON et al., 1966; SHORTER et al., 1968, 1969).

Crohn's disase: The problems concerning immunologic reactions in Crohn's disease are more difficult. Crohn's disease of the colon (granulomatous colitis) seems to be immunologically identical to ulcerative colitis (THAYER et al., 1969; GINSBERG, 1971). With regard to the difficult and often contradictory results in so-called regional enteritis we may refer to the literature (SHORTER et al., 1969; BROOKE et al., 1969; JONES et al., 1969; SØLTOFT, 1969, 1970; EGGERT et al., 1969; BENDIXEN, 1969, 1971; GEFFROY et al., 1970, 1971).

While pathologic immune and autoimmune reactions in the course of idiopathic steatorrhoea, ulcerative proctocolitis, and Crohn's disease are proved, there still remains the question of whether this immune response is a primary

or a secondary one. There is much morphologic evidence that the interepithelial
lymphocytes whose cytoarchitecture corresponds to those of lymphocytes
whose cytoarchitecture corresponds to those of lymphocytes stimulated by
Phythaemagglutinin are concerned with the immune reactions. All stimulation
and proliferation of the so-called peripheral lymphoid system (NOSSAL, 1969)
depends, however, on the antigenic stimulus.

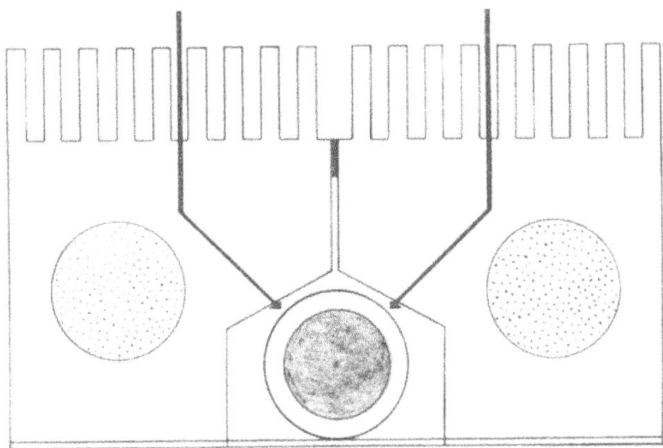

Fig. 13. Schematic diagram of the position of interepithelial lymphocytes. Arrows are
pointing in the main direction of absorbed substances

Apparently the interepithelial lymphocytes are also a heterogenous group
of cells with regard to function, comparable to those of the circulating pool
and the lymphoid organs or tissues. In theory the following functional differentiations are possible:

1. *Memory cells* which according to GOWANS and UHR (1966) and ELLIS
et al. (1969) increase in size and proliferate after having been stimulated by
immunogenes for the second time;

2. *"Antigen-reactive cells"* (see also NOSSAL, 1968, 1969; NOSSAL *et al.*,
1965): MILLER and MITCHEL (1968) and NOSSAL *et al.* (1968) assume some
antigens provoking immunologic reactions involving two cell-populations:
1. the so-called antigen-reactive cells and 2. precursors of antibody producing
cells. After reacting with the antigenic substance, the antigen-reactive cells
promote the transformation of precursors of antibody-producing cells. On the
basis of their special position within the interepithelial space (see also Fig. 13),
interepithelial lymphocytes may have this antigen reactivity;

3. *"Nurse cells"* respectively *"carrier specific cells"* (MITCHISON, 1967,
1969, 1970): Experimental studies on animals with regard to the interaction
of lymphocytes have shown that there is a cooperation between hapten-specific
and carrier-specific cells, the latter having a so-called nurse function in the
immune response. It is possible that the only task of these nurse cells is to
concentrate antigenic substances and to transfer them in adequate form to

antibody-producing cells. But apparently there is no general difference between antigen-reactive and carrier-specific cells. Both the position in the epithelial layer and the intimate contact with the lateral wall of the adjacent epithelial cells predispose the interepithelial lymphocytes to both functions.

The intestinal epithelial cells have a polar apico-basal differentation. The significance of this for the passage of substances is that there is transcellular unipolar transport (see also Fig. 13). In the apical region substrates are ingested by the cell partly by pinocytosis and micropinocytosis, partly by active directed absorption across the cell membrane. The ingested substrates are moved towards the sides of the cell into extracellular spaces (DIAMOND and TORMEY, 1966; CARDELL *et al.*, 1967; DAVID *et al.*, 1967; IMAI and COULSTON, 1968; HERZER *et al.*, 1969, 1970; AMON, 1969; GARDNER *et al.*, 1970) and from there they enter the bloodstream and lymphatic system. Within these lateral spaces the interepithelial lymphocytes are now in an ideal position where they can come into contact with antigenic substances as antigen-reactive cells (Fig. 13);

4. *"Cytotoxic, aggressive, lymphocytes:* The lymphocytic cytotoxicity plays an important part in versus host reactions (References: GRUNDMANN, 1970). In epidermal transplantations the lymphocytes are very close to epidermal cells before the rejection necrosis is seen (WIENER *et al.*, 1964). Because of this special position a cytotoxic effect has been attributed to these lymphocytes (WAKSMAN, 1963, 1964). FISCHER *et al.* (1969) that demonstrated by impressively activyted lymphocytes ("effector cells") are able to destroy the so-called target cells by repeated contact. Apparently even a few immunologically active cells are enough to destroy a homeo-transplant. Probably the so-called "migration inhibitory factor" is essential in this process (DAVID, 1966; BLOOM and BENNETT, 1966).

Lymphocytes cytotoxic to allogenic epithelial cells of the colon have been demonstrated by WATSON *et al.* (1966) and SHORTER *et al.* (1968, 1969). This apparently colon-specific cytotoxic effect can also be produced by incubation of lymphocytes with a lipopolysaccharide extract from Escherichia coli 01 19 B14. There seems to be a close similarity between the antigens of the colonic epithelial cells and the bacteria of the gut. WATSON and BOLT (1968) propose that the immunologic process in ulcerative colitis is probably of a cellular type, which is primarily directed against bacterial lipopolysaccharides, these therefore being the true antigen (see also WATSON, 1969a, b). But because of the above-mentioned similarity between both antigens the epithelial cells of the colon also become target cells.

There is evidence that some interepithelial lymphocytes are involved in these cellular reactions, the bacterial lipopolysaccharides, lateral space and interepithelial lymphocytes engaging in a continuous series of reactions.

As early as 1932 WATZKA reported deep effective alterations in the epithelial cells in close proximity to lymphocytes. These alterations can be generally regarded as a dedifferentiation and a step of regression to an anaplastic state (see also Fig. 14).

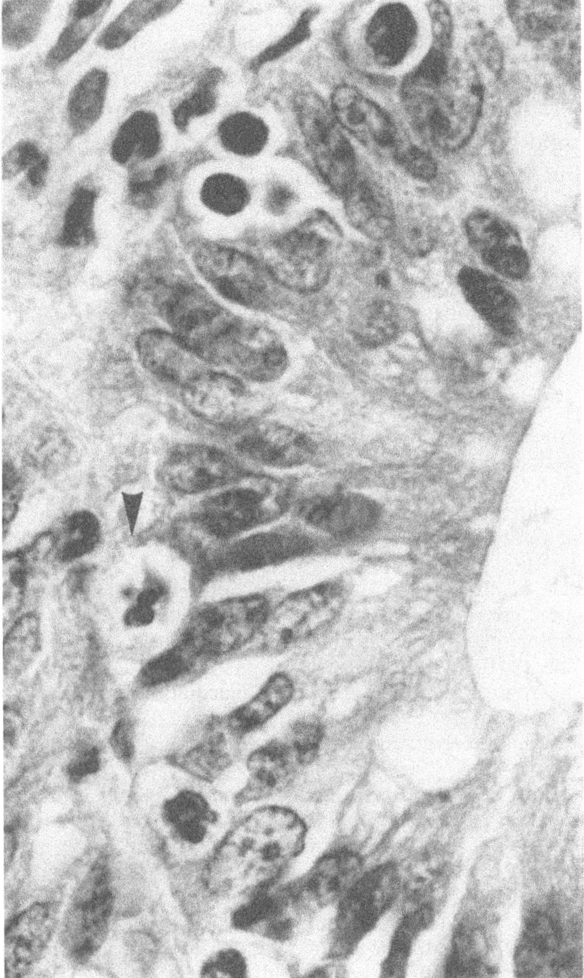

Fig. 14. Light micrograph of mucous membrane of the colon from a patient with active ulcerative colitis. Numerous lymphocytes between irritable, dark basophilia columnar cells. Magn. 1 500 ×

VI. Conclusions

The problems concerning interepithelial lymphocytes, especially their function, still remain unsolved. Nevertheless there are a number of results that mark them as immunocompetent cells. The functional differentiations have been discussed from the theoretical standpoint. There seems to be no doubt that according to the comprehensive definition of MEDAWAR (1960, 1965) the interepithelial lymphocytes have an immunological competence. Any conclusions going beyond this are speculative.

There are a number of inconsistent findings. For example there should be at least a small number of activated interepithelial lymphocytes corresponding to the "low grade response" postulated by TONER et al. (1971).

The morphologic results are very contradictory in this field, especially those obtained by electron microscopy (Toner *et al.*, 1971; Otto and Martin, 1971; Otto and Walke, 1972; Walke, 1972). More satisfactory interpretations might be possible if membrane-fixed receptor structures of the interepithelial lymphocytes could be demonstrated. Especially the methods of micropunction and of recording bioelectric potentials of epithelial cells and interepithelial lymphocytes should give more insight.

The hypothesis of the biologically, active symbiosis between interepithelial lymphocytes and epithelial cells discussed above could non be verified from an immunologic viewpoint.

References

Ackerman, G. A.: Electron microscopy of the bursa of Fabricius of the embryonic chick with particular reference to the lympho-epithelial nodules. J. Cell Biol. **13**, 127–146 (1962).

Afzelius, B. A.: The nucleus of Noctiluca Scintillans. Aspects of nucleocytoplasmic exchanges and the formation of nuclear membrane. J. Cell Biol. **19**, 229–238 (1963).

Alarcon-Segovia, D., Herskovic, T., Wakim, K. G., Green, P. A., Scudamore, H. H.: Presence of circulating antibodies to gluten and milk fractions in patients with non-tropical sprue. Amer. J. Med. **36**, 485–499 (1964).

Amon, H.: Morphologische Kriterien von Resorptions- und Exkretionsvorgängen. Med. Welt (N. F.) **20**, 1371–1378 (1969).

Andrew, W.: The role of lymphocytes in the normal epidermis. Anat. Rec. **103**, 419 (1949).

Andrew, W.: Lymphocyte transformation in epithelium. J. nat. Cancer Inst. **35**, 113–137 (1965).

Andrew, W., Andrew, N. V.: Mitotic division and degeneration of lymphocytes within the cells of intestinal epithelium in the mouse. Anat. Rec. **93**, 251–277 (1945).

Andrew, W., Andrew, N. V.: Lymphocytes in the normal epidermis of the rat and of man. Anat. Rec. **104**, 217–232 (1949).

Andrew, W., Collings, C. K.: Lymphocytes within the cells of intestinal epithelium in man. Anat. Rec. **96**, 445–457 (1946).

Andrew, W., Sosa, J. M.: Mitotic division and degeneration of lymphocytes within cells of intestinal epithelium in young and adult white mice. Anat. Rec. **97**, 63–98 (1947).

Arnstein, C. von: Über Becherzellen und ihre Beziehung zur Fettresorption und Sekretion. Arch. mikr. Anat. **39**, 527–547 (1867).

Asheron, G. L., Broberger, O.: Incidence of hemagglutinating and complement-fixing antibodies. Brit. med. J. **1961**I, 1429–1433.

Asquith, P., Thompson, R. A., Cooke, W. T.: Serumimmunoglobulins in adult coelic disease. Lancet **1969**II, 129–131.

Astaldi, G., Airo, R., Conrad, M. E., Penna, R., Ceretto, F.: Lymphatic follicles and immunologic cell reaction in human jejunal mucosa obtained by peroral biopsy in infectious hepatitis. In: Lymphatic tissue and germinal centers in immune response. New York, Washington, London: Plenum Press 1969.

Astaldi, G., Conrad, M. E., Airo, R.: Mast cells in the normal human jejunum: a comparison with specimens obtained during infectious hepatitis. Amer. J. dig. Dis. **11**, 53–62 (1966).

Béguin, F.: L'intestin pendant le jeune et l'intestin pendant la digestion. Etudes faites sur le Crapaud des joncs et le Lézard des murailles. Arch. Anat. micr. Morph. exp. **6**, 385–454 (1904).

Bendixen, G.: Cellular hypersensitivity to components of intestinal mucosa in ulcerative colitis and Crohn's disease. Gut **10**, 631–636 (1969).

Bendixen, G.: Cellular hypersensitivity in ulcerative colitis and Crohn's disease. Schweiz. med. Wschr. **101**, 698–701 (1971).

BERKE, G., GINSBURG, H., FELDMAN, M.: Graft reaction in tissue culture.3. Effect of phytohaemagglutinin. Immunology 16, 659–667 (1969).
BILLINGHAM, R. E., SPARROW, E. M.: Studies on the nature of immunity to homologous grafted skin, with special reference to the use pure epidermal grafts. J. exp. Biol. 31, 16–39 (1954).
BLECHER, T. E., AJDUKIEWICZ, A. B., McCARTHY, C. F., READ, A. E.: Serum immunoglobulins and lymphocyte transformation studies in coelic disease. Gut 10, 57–62 (1969).
BLOOM, B. R., BENNETT, B.: Mechanism of a reaction in vitro associated with delayed-type hypersensitivity. Science 153, 80–82 (1966).
BLOOM, B. R., BENNETT, B.: Migration inhibitory factor associated with delayedtype hypersensitivity. Fed. Proc. 27, 13–15 (1968).
BLOOM, G. D.: Structural and biochemical characteristics of mast cells. In: The inflammatory process. New York: Academic Press, Inc. 1965.
BOHLE, A., HAUSSMANN, P., VOGT, W.: Über Beziehungen zwischen Lymphozyten und Harnkanälchenepithelien in der Niere des Menschen. Klin. Wschr. 48, 1323–1326 (1970).
BOS, W. H.: Recirculatie en transformatie van lymphocyten. Groningen: Drukkerij van Denderen 1967.
BOURNE, F. J., PICKUP, J., HONOUR, J. W.: Intestinal immunoglobulins in the pig. Biochim. biophys. Acta (Amst.) 229, 18–25 (1971).
BRAUS, H.: Anatomie des Menschen, 1. Aufl. Berlin: Springer 1924.
BREGMAN, E., KIRSNER, J. B.: Colon antibodies in ulcerative colitis. J. Lab. clin. Med. 56, 785 (1960).
BRINKMAN, G. L.: The mast cell in normal human bronchus and lung. J. Ultrastruct. Res. 23, 115–123 (1968).
BROBERGER, O., PERLMANN, P.: Autoantibodies in human ulcerative colitis. J. exp. Med. 110, 657–674 (1959).
BROOKE, B. N., HOFFMANN, D. C., SWARBRICK, E. T.: Azathioprine for Crohn's disease. Lancet 1969 II, 612–614.
BROWN, D. L., COOPER, A. G., HEPNER, G. W.: IgM metabolism in coeliac disease. Lancet 1969 I, 858–861.
BRUNNER, K. T., MANUEL, J., CEROTTINI, J. C.: Quantitative assay of the lytic action of immune lymphoid cells on 51-Cr-labelled allogeneis target cells in vitro; inhibition by isoantibody and by drugs. Immunology 14, 181–196 (1968).
BRUNNER, K. T., MANUEL, J., SCHINDLER, R.: Inhibitory effect of isoantibody on in vivo sensitization and on the in vitro cytotoxic action of immune lymphocytes. Nature (Lond.) 213, 1246–1247 (1967).
BRYANT, B. J.: Reutilization on leukocyte DNA by cells of regenerating liver. Exp. Cell Res. 27, 70–79 (1962).
CARDELL, R. R., BADENHAUSEN, S., PORTER, K. R.: Intestinal triglyceride absorption in the rat. An electron microscopical study. J. Cell Biol. 34, 123–155 (1967).
CARR, K. E.: Fine structure of crystalline inclusions in the globule leucocyte of the mouse intestine. J. Anat. (Lond.) 101, 793–803 (1967).
CARR, K. E., WHUR, P.: Ultrastructure of globule leucocyte inclusions in the rat and mouse. Z. Zellforsch. 86, 153–162 (1968).
CARREL, A.: Leukocytic trephones. J. Amer. med. Ass. 82, 255–258 (1924).
CLAWSON, C. C., COOPER, M. D., GOOD, R. A.: Lymphocyte fine structure in the bursa of Fabricius, the thymus, and the germinal centers. Lab. Invest. 16, 407–421 (1967).
CORNELIUS, W.: Contribution à l'étude clinique et expérimentale de la recto-colite hémorrhagique. Mémoires assistant étranger, Faculté Medicine, Paris 1958.
CORTI, A.: Granulazioni e fatti morfocinetici delle cellule mononucleate migranti nell' epithelio del villo intestinale di mammiferi. Biologica (Torino) 1, 1–27 (1907).
CORTI, A.: Contributo alla determinazione specifica delle cellule mononucleato migranti nell'epithelio intestinale ed allo studio delle loro funzioni. Haematologica (Palermo) 3, 121–150 (1922).
COTTIER, H., BÜRKI, H., BÜRKI, K., LAISSUE, J.: Mit Bildung humoraler Antikörper einhergehende Immunreaktionen: Die anamnestische Reizbeantwortung. In: Handbuch der allgemeinen Pathologie, Bd. VII/3. Berlin-Heidelberg-New York: Springer 1970.

Cottier, H., Hess, M. W., Roos, B., Grétillat, P. A.: Regeneration, Hyperplasie und Onkogenese der lymphoretikulären Organe. In: Handbuch der allgemeinen Pathologie, Bd. VI/2. Berlin-Heidelberg-New York: Springer 1969.

Cottier, H., Hess, M. W., Roos, B., Sordat, B.: Die zellulären Grundlagen der immunobiologischen Reizbeantwortung. Verh. dtsch. Ges. Path. 54, 1–27 (1970).

Dameshek, W.: "Immunoblasts" and "immunocytes" — an attempt at a functional nomenclature. Blood 21, 243–245 (1963).

Darcy, D. A.: A study of the plasma cell and lymphocyte in rabbit tissue homografts. Phil. Trans. B 236, 463–503 (1952).

Darlington, D., Rogers, A. W.: Epithelial lymphocytes in the small intestine of the mouse. J. Anat. Lond.)(100, 813–830 (1966).

David, H., Lisewski, G., Marx, I.: Zur Problematik der Resorptionsstörungen bei chronischer Enteritis (ein Beitrag zur Pathogenese des Malabsorptionssyndroms). Dtsch. Gesundh.-Wes. 22, 385–395 (1967).

David, J. R.: Delayed hypersensitivity in vitro: its mediation by cell-free substances formed by lymphoid cell-antigen interaction. Proc. nat. Acad. Sci. (Wash.) 56, 72–77 (1966).

Davidoff, M. von: Untersuchungen über die Beziehungen des Darmepithels zum lymphoiden Gewebe. Arch. mikr. Anat. 29, 495–525 (1887).

Diamond, J. M., McD. Tormey, J.: Role of long extracellular channels in fluid transport across epithelia. Nature (Lond.) 210, 817–820 (1966).

Dobbins, W. O., Tomasini, J. T., Emory, L.: Electron and light microscopic identification of the mast cell of the gastrointestinal tract. Gastroenterology 56, 268–279 (1969).

Doerr, W.: Über lymphoepitheliale Geschwülste Schmincke-Regaud. Ärztl. Wschr. 11, 169–182 (1956).

Dresser, D. W.: Adjuvanticity of vitamin A. Nature (Lond.) 217, 527–529 (1968).

Dresser, D. W.: An assay for adjuvanticity. Clin. exp. Immunol. 3, 877–888 (1968).

Eberth, J.: Zur Entstehung der Schleimkörper. Virchows Arch. path. Anat. 21, 106–115 (1861).

Eberth, J.: Über den feineren Bau der Darmschleimhaut. Würzburg. Naturwiss. Z. 5, 23–33 (1864).

Edinger, L.: Über die Schleimhaut des Fischdarmes nebst Bemerkungen zur Phylogenese der Drüsen des Darmrohres Arch. mikr. Anat. 13, 651–692 (1877).

Eggert, R. C.: Die Wege des Fettes in der Darmschleimhaut bei seiner Resportion. Virchows Arch. path. Anat. 48, 119–176 (1869).

Eggert, R. C.: Neue und alte Mitteilungen über Fettresorption im Dünndarm und im Dickdarm. Biol. Zbl. 4, 580–600 (1884).

Eggert, R. C., Wilson, I. D., Good, R. A.: Agammaglobulinemia and regional enteritis. Ann. intern. Med. 71, 581–585 (1969).

Eimer, Th.: Zur Fettresorption und zur Entstehung der Schleim- und Eiterkörperchen. Virchows Arch. path. Anat. 38, 428–432 (1866).

Ellis, S. T., Gowans, J. L., Howard, J. C.: The origin of antibody forming cells from lymphocytes. Antibiot. et Chemother. (Basel) 15, 40–55 (1969).

Everett, N. B., Caffrey, R. W., Rieke, W. O.: Recirculation of lymphocytes. Ann. N.Y. Acad. Sci. 113, 887–897 (1964).

Fagraeus, A.: Antibody production in relation to the development of plasma cells: in vivo and in vitro experiments. Acta med. scand. 204, Suppl., 1–122 (1948).

Fagraeus, A.: Nomenclature of immunologically competent cells. In: Ciba Foundation Symposium on Cellular Aspects of Immunity. London: Churchill 1960.

Farquhar, M. G., Palade, G. E.: Junctional complexes in various epithelia. J. Cell Biol. 17, 375–412 (1963).

Fawcett, D. W.: The membranes of the cytoplasm. Lab. Invest. 10, 1162–1188 (1961).

Fedorko, M. E., Hirsch, J. G.: Crystalloid structure in granules of guinea pig basophils and human mast cells. J. Cell Biol. 26, 973–976 (1965).

Fichtelius, K. E.: The mammalian equivalent to Bursa Fabricii of birds. Exp. Cell Res. 46, 231–234 (1967).

Fichtelius, K. E.: The gut epithelium — a first level lymphoid organ? Exp. Cell Res. 49, 87–104 (1968).

FICHTELIUS, K. E., FINSTAD, J., GOOD, R. A.: The phylogenetic occurence of lymphocytes within the gut epithelium. Int. Arch. Allergy 35, 119–133 (1969a).

FICHTELIUS, K. E., JAROSLOW, B. N.: Changes in the concentration of lymphocytes in the intestinal epithelium of hibernating ground squirrels (Citellus Tridecemlineatus). Acta path. microbiol. scand. 77, 99–102 (1969).

FICHTELIUS, K. E., SUNDSTRÖM, C., KULLGREN, B., LINNA, J.: The lympho-epithelial organs of homo sapiens revisited. Acta path. microbiol. scand. 77, 103–116 (1969b).

FINSTAD, J., GOOD, R. A.: Phylogenetic studies of adaptive immune responses in the lower vertebrates. In: Phylogeny of immunity. Gainesville: University of Florida Press 1966.

FISCHER, H., AX, W., MALCHOW, H., ZEISS, I.: Studies on the cytotoxicity of lymphocytes. Current Problems in Immunology. Bayer-Symposium I, 113–120 (1969).

FISCHER, H., RÜDE, E., SELLIN, D.: Membranaspekte der Immunologie. Naturwissenschaften 57, 507–513 (1970).

GARDNER, J. D., BROWN, M. S., LASTER, L.: The columnar epithelial cell of the small intestine: digestion and transport. New Engl. J. Med. 283, 1196–1202; 1264–1271; 1317–1324 (1970).

GEFFROY, Y., COLIN, R., CHARVET, PH.: Essai de traitement immunologique de la maladie de Crohn. Arch. Mal. Appar. dig. 59, 157–162 (1970).

GEFFROY, Y., COLIN, R., HECKETSWEILER, PH.: Aspects nouveaux du traitement de la maladie de Crohn. Rev. Prat. (Paris) 21, 2599–2612 (1971).

GELZAYD, E. A., KRAFT, S. C., KIRSNER, J. B.: Distribution of immunoglobulins in human rectal mucosa. Gastroenterology 54, 334–340 (1968).

GINSBERG, A. L.: Alterations in immunologic mechanisms in disease of the gastrointestinal tract. Dig. Dis. 16, 61–80 (1971).

GLIMSTEDT, E. G.: Nagra nya rön baserade pa jämförelse mellan sterilt uppfödda djur och kontrolldjur. Med. För. Tidskrift 11, 271–277 (1933).

GOLDNER, J.: Le problème de la régénération de l'épithélium intestinal. Bull. Histol. appl. 6, 79–95 (1929).

GOOD, R. A., FINSTAD, J., POLLARA, B., GABRIELSEN, A. E.: Morphologic studies on the evolution of lymphoid tissues among lower vertebrates. In: Phylogeny of immunity. Gainesville: University of Florida Press 1966.

GOOD, R. A., PAPERMASTER, B. W.: Ontogeny and phylogenyo f adaptive immunity. Adv. Immunol. 4, 1–115 (1964).

GOWANS, J. L., McGREGOR, D. D.: The immunological activities of lymphocytes. Progr. Allergy 9, 1–78 (1965).

GOWANS, J. L., McGREGOR, D. D., COWEN, D. M., FORD, C. E.: Initiation of immune responses by small lymphocytes. Nature (Lond.) 196, 651–655 (1962).

GOWANS, J. L., UHR, J. W.: The carriage of immunological memory by small lymphocytes in the rat. J. exp. Med. 124, 1017–1030 (1966).

GRUNDMANN, E.: Die Immunopathologie der experimentellen Allo- und Xenotransplantation. Verh. dtsch. Ges. Path. 54, 65–94 (1970).

GUIEYSSE-PELLISSIER, A.: Etude sur la structure du noyau des cellules épithéliales de l'intestin de Scyllium catulus. C. R. Soc. Biol. (Paris) 71, 553–555 (1911).

GUIEYSSE-PELLISSIER, A.: Caryoanabiose et greffe nucléaire. Arch. Anat. micr. Morph. exp. 13, 1–54 (1912).

HALL, J. G., SMITH, M. E.: Homing lymph-borne immunoblasts to the gut. Nature (Lond.) 226, 262–263 (1970).

HARRIS, O. D., COOKE, W. T., THOMPSON, H., WATERHOUSE, J. A. H.: Malignancy in adult coeliac disease and idiopathic steatorrhea. Amer. J. Med. 42, 899–912 (1967).

HARTMANN, A.: Neuere Untersuchungen über den lymphoiden Apparat des Kaninchendarmes. Anat. Anz. 47, 65–90 (1914).

HAYWARD, A. F., FRESTON, J. W., BOUCHIER, I. A.: Changes in the ultrastructure of gall bladder epithelium in rabbits with experimental gallstones. Gut 9, 550–556 (1968).

HEBEL, R., LIEBICH, H.-G.: Elektronenmikroskopische Untersuchungen an kleinen Lymphozyten aus dem Ductus thoracicus der Ratte. Z. Zellforsch. 93, 232–248 (1969).

HEIDENHAIN, R.: Beiträge zur Histologie und Physiologie der Dünndarmschleimhaut. Pflügers Arch. ges. Physiol. 43, Suppl., 1–103 (1888).

HELLMAN, T.: Die Einlagerung von Zellen in Schleimhäuten und Epithel. Antwort an J. SOBOTTA. Anat. Anz. 78, 65–68 (1934).

Hermans, P. E.: Nodular lymphoid hyperplasia of the small intestine and hypo-gamma-globulinemia: Theoretical and proctical considerations. Fed. Proc. **26**, 1606–1611 (1967).

Herskovic, T., Katz, J., Gryboski, J. D.: Coproantibodies to gluten in celiac disease. J. Amer. med. Ass. **203**, 887–888 (1968).

Herzer, R., Merker, H. J., Dennhardt, R., Haberich, F. J.: Resorptions- und Sekretionsstudien am Darm. 4. Mitt.: Die Bedeutung der Intercellularspalten für den Nettoflüßigkeitstransport am Dickdarm mit gleichzeitigem histochemischen Nachweis von ATPase (Rattenversuche). Z. ges. exp. Med. **152**, 8–19 (1970).

Herzer, R., Merker, H. J., Haberich, F. J.: Resorptions- und Sekretionsstudien am Darm. 3. Mitt.: Die Bedeutung der Intercellularspalten für den Nettoflüßigkeitstransport am Dünndarm (Rattenversuche). Z. ges. exp. Med. **150**, 239–250 (1969).

Hess, M. W.: Lymphatischer Apparat, insbesondere Thymus, in der Pathogenese der Defektimmunopathien. In: Handbuch der allgemeinen Pathologie, Bd. VII/3. Berlin-Heidelberg-New York: Springer 1970.

Hessling, Th. von: Grundzüge der allgemeinen und speziellen Gewebelehre des Menschen. Leipzig 1866.

Hobbs, J. R., Hepner, G. W., Douglas, A. P., Crabbé, P. A., Johansson, S. G. O.: Immunological mystery of coeliac disease. Lancet **1969** II, 649–650.

Housley, J., Asquith, P., Cooke, W. T.: Immune response to gluten in adult coeliac disease. Brit. med. J. **1969** I, 159–161.

Humble, J. G., Jayne, W. H. W., Pulvertaft, R. J. V.: Biological interaction between lymphocytes and other cells. Brit. J. Haemat. **2**, 283–294 (1956).

Hurlimann, J.: Immunoglobulin synthesis and transport by human salivary glands. Immunological mechanisms of the mucous membranes. Curr. Top. Pathol. **55**, 69–108 (1971).

Imai, H., Coulston, F.: Ultrastructural studies of absorption of methoxychlor in the jejunal mucosa of the rat. Exp. molec. Path. **8**, 135–158 (1968).

Immonen, P., Kouvalainen, K., Visakorpi, J. K.: The immunoelectrophoretic gamma-A globulin in malabsorption. Ann. paediat. (Basel) **207**, 269–276 (1966).

Jassinowsky, M. A.: Über die Emigration auf den Schleimhäuten des Verdauungskanals. Frankfurt. Z. Path. **32**, 238–244 (1925).

Jolly, J.: Cited by Watzka, M.: Verh. anat. Ges. (Jena) **41**, 150–158 (1932).

Jones, J. V., Housley, J., Ashurst, P. M., Hawkins, C. F.: Development of delayed hypersensitivity to dinitrochlorbenzenein patients with Crohn's disease. Gut **10**, 52–56 (1969).

Katz, J., Kantor, F. S., Herskovic, T.: Intestinal antibodies to wheat fractions in coeliac disease. Ann. intern. Med. **69**, 1149–1153 (1968).

Kellas, L. M.: An intra-epithelial granular cell in the uterine epithelium of some ruminant species during the pregnancy cycle. Acta anat. (Basel) **44**, 109–130 (1961).

Kelsall, M. A.: Lymphocytes in the intestinal epithelium and Peyer's pathces of normal and tumorbearing hamsters. Anat. Rec. **96**, 391–409 (1946).

Kelsall, M. A., Crabb, E. D.: Lymphocytes and plasmocytes in nucleoprotein metabolism. Ann. N.Y. Acad. Sci. **72**, 295–337 (1958).

Kelsall, M. A., Crabb, E. D.: Lymphocytes and mast cells. Baltimore. Williams and Wilkins 1959.

Kent, J. F.: The origin, fate and cytochemistry of the globule leucocyte of the sheep. Anat. Rec. **112**, 91–115 (1952).

Kent, J. F.: Distribution and fine structure of globule leucocytes in respiratory and digestive tracts of the laboratory rat. Anat. Rec. **156**, 439–453 (1966).

Kessel, R. G.: An electron microscope study of nuclear-cytoplasmic exchange in oocytes of Ciona intestinalis. J. Ultrastruct. Res. **15**, 181–196 (1966).

Kirkman, H.: A comparative morphological and cytochemical study of globule leucocytes (Schollen-Leukozyten) of the urinary tract, and of possibly related cells. Amer. J. Anat. **86**, 91–131 (1950).

Kivel, R. M., Kearns, D. H., Liebowitz, D.: Significance of antibodies to dietary proteins in the serum of patients with nontropical sprue. New Engl. J. Med. **271**, 769–772 (1964).

Klein, E., Klein, G., Nadkarni, J. S.: Surface IgM-kappa specificity on a Burkitt lymphoma cell in vivo and in derived culture lines. Cancer Res. **28**, 1300–1310 (1968).

Koelliker, A.: Handbuch der Gewebelehre des Menschen, 5. Aufl. Leipzig 1867.

KÖLSCH, E., MITCHISON, N. A.: The subcellular distribution of antigens in macrophages. J. exp. Med. **128**, 1059–1079 (1968).

KOTANI, M., YAMASHITA, A., RAI, F., SEIKI, K., HORRII, I.: Reutilization of DNA breakdown products from lymphocytes in lumen of intestine. Blood **29**, Suppl. 616–627 (1967).

LAGERCRANTZ, R., HAMMARSTRÖM, S., PERLMANN, P., GUSTAFSSON, B. E.: Immunological studies in ulcerative colitis. IV. Origin of autoantibodies. J. exp. Med. **128**, 1339–1352 (1968).

LAGUENS, R., SCHAPOSNIK, F., ECHEVERRIA, R., CALAFELL, R., CONTI, A.: Fine structure of the small bowel in dermatitis herpetiformis. Virchows Arch. Abt. A **352**, 34–42 (1971).

LEHNER, T.: Pathology of recurrent oral ulceration and oral ulceration in Behcet's syndrome. Light electron and fluorescence microscopy. J. Path. Bact. **97**, 481–494 (1969).

LE PORE, M. J.: Long-term or maintenance adrenal steroid therapy in nontropical sprue. Amer. J. Med. **25**, 381–390 (1958).

LEVIN, A. G., FRIBERG, S., JR., KLEIN, E.: Xenotransplantation of a Burkitt lymphoma culture line with surface immunoglobulin specificity. Nature (Lond.) **222**, 997–998 (1969).

LEWIS, W. H.: Locomotion of lymphocytes. Bull. Johns Hopk. Hosp. **49**, 29–36 (1931).

LIPSKY, A.: Beiträge zur Kenntnis des feineren Baues des Darmkanales. S.-B. Akad. Wiss. Wien., math.-nat. Kl. **55**, 183–192 (1867).

LOEWENSTEIN, W. R.: Cell surface membranes in close contact. Role of calcium and magnesium ions. J. Colloid. Interface Sci. **25**, 34–46 (1967).

LOEWENSTEIN, W. R.: Transfer of information through cell junctions and growth control. Canad. Cancer Conf. **8**, 162–170 (1969).

LOEWENSTEIN, W. R., KANNO, Y.: Studies on an epithelial (gland) cell junction. I. Modifications of surface membrane permeability. J. Cell Biol. **22**, 565–586 (1964).

LOEWENSTEIN, W. R., NAKAS, M., SOCOLAR, S. J.: Junctional membrane uncoupling. Permeability transformations at a cell membrane junctions. J. gen. Physiol. **50**, 1865–1891 (1967).

LOW, F. N., FREEMAN, J. A.: Electron microscopic atlas of normal and leukemic human blood. New York: McGraw Hill 1958.

MARKS, J., SHUSTER, S., WATSON, A. J.: Small bowel changes in dermatitis herpetiformis. Lancet **1966II**, 1280–1282.

MARKS, J., WHITE, M. W., BEARD, R. J., ROBERTSON, W. B., GOLD, S. C.: Small bowel abnormalities in dermatitis herpetiformis. Brit. med. J. **1968I**, 552–555.

MARSHALL, A. H. E., WHITE, R. G.: Reactions of the reticular tissues to antigens. Brit. J. exp. Path. **31**, 157–174 (1950).

MEADER, R. D., LANDERS, D. F.: Electron and light microscopic observations on relationship between lymphocytes and intestinal epithelium. Amer. J. Anat. **121**, 763–774 (1967).

MEDAWAR, P. B.: Theories of immunological tolerance. In: Ciba Foundation Symposium on Cellular Aspects of Immunity. London: Churchill 1960.

MEDAWAR, P. B.: Introduction to: transplantation of tissue and organs. Brit. med. Bull. **21**, 97–99 (1965).

MIETENS, C.: Untersuchungen über Antikörperbildung gegen Gliadin und Milchproteine. I. Die Bildung komplementbindender Antikörper bei Patienten mit Coeliakie und anderen intestinalen Erkrankungen sowie bei gesunden Kontrollkindern. Z. Kinderheilk. **98**, 254–267 (1967a).

MIETENS, C.: Untersuchungen über Antikörperbildung gegen Gliadin und Milchproteine. II. Der Nachweis von M durch Ultrazentrifugation und Behandlung mit Mercaptoäthanol. Z. Kinderheilk. **99**, 130–139 (1967b).

MIETENS, C., JOHANSSON, S. G. O., BENNICH, H.: Serumkonzentrationen der Immunoglobuline bei Kindern im Verlauf der Cöliakie unter besonderer Berücksichtigung von IgE. Klin. Wschr. **49**, 256–260 (1971).

MILLER, J. F. A., MITCHELL, G. F.: Cell to cell interaction in the immune response. I. Hemolysin-forming cells in neonatally thymectomized mice reconstituted with thymus or thoracic duct lymphocytes. J. exp. Med. **128**, 801–820 (1968).

Mitchison, N. A.: Antigen recognition responsible for the induction in vitro of the secondary response. Cold Spr. Harb. Symp. quant. Biol. 32, 431–439 (1967).

Mitchison, N. A.: Unmasking of cell-associated foreign antigen during incubation of lymphoid cells. Israel J. med. Sci. 5, 230–234 (1969).

Mitchison, N. A.: Cellular and molecular recognition mechanism prior to the immune response. In: Handbuch der allgemeinen Pathologie, Bd. VII/3. Berlin-Heidelberg-New York: Springer 1970.

Mollier, S.: Die lymphoepithelialen Organe. 5. Ber. d. Ges. f. Morphol. u. Physiol., München 1913.

Monti, R.: La funzione di secrezione e di assorbimento intestinale studiate negli animale ibernanti. Mem. letta al R. inst. Lomb. Pavia 1903.

Mori, Y., Lennert, K.: Electron microscopic atlas of lymph node cytology and pathology. Berlin-Heidelberg-New York: Springer 1969.

Murray, M., Miller, H. R. P., Jarrett, W. F. H.: The globule leukocyte and its derivation from the subepithelial mast cell. Lab. Invest. 19, 222–234 (1968).

Muthmann, E.: Beiträge zur vergleichenden Anatomie der Blinddärme und der lymphoiden Organe des Darmkanals bei Säugetieren und Vögeln. Anat. H. 48, 65–114 (1913).

Nakano, A.: Über die Zahl der Wanderzellen in der Darmschleimhaut und die Correlation zwischen der Wanderzellenzahl und dem lymphatischen Apparat der Darmwand und insbesondere der Noduli lymphatici aggregati, 1929. Ref. Jap. J. med. Sci., Trans. Anat. 3, Nr 115, 1 (1931).

Nemetschek-Gansler, H., Wagner, A.: Morphologischer und klinischer Beitrag zu den Enteropathien. Dünndarmbiopsien. Virchows Arch. Abt. A 346, 154–167 (1969).

Nossal, G. J. V.: The cellular basis of immunity. Presented as: The Harvey Lecture, March 1968 at the New York Academy of Medicine.

Nossal, G. J. V.: Die Regulation der Immunantwort. Klin. Wschr. 47, 568–573 (1969).

Nossal, G. J. V., Abbot, A., Mitchell, J., Lummus, Z.: Antigens in immunity. XV. Ultrastructural features of antigen capture in primary and secondary lymphoid follicles. J. exp. Med. 127, 277–290 (1968).

Nossal, G. J. V., Ada, G. L., Austin, C. M.: Antigens in immunity. IX. The antigen content of single antibody-forming cells. J. exp. Med. 121, 945–954 (1965).

Nossal, G. J. V., Mäkelä, O.: Autoradiographic studies on the immune response. I. The kinetics of plasma cell proliferation. J. exp. Med. 115, 209–230 (1962).

Nossal, G. J. V., Mitchell, J.: The nature of RNA synthesis in immune induction. In: Immunopathology, 3rd International Symposium. Basel and Stuttgart: Schwalbe & Co. 1963.

Oppel, A.: Über den Darm der Monotremen, einiger Marsupialier und von Manis javanica. Zool. Forsch.reisen 2, 403–433 (1897).

Otto, H. F.: Über Beobachtungen zum kompletten Paneth-Zellschwund bei idiopathischer Steatorrhoe. Beitr. Path. 143, 378–389 (1971a).

Otto, H. F.: Not published (1971b).

Otto, H. F., Martin, W.: Zur cytologischen Ultrastruktur des Schleimhautstroma bei Enteropathien, insbesondere bei der idiopathischen Steatorrhoe. Virchows Arch. Abt. A 353, 191–206 (1971).

Otto, H. F., Walke, A.: Über lympho-epitheliale Beziehungen bei Enteropathien. Virchows Arch. Abt. A 355, 85–98 (1972).

Otto, H. F., Weitz, H.: Elektronenmikroskopische Untersuchungen an Paneth-Zellen der Ratte unter zinkarmer Diät. Beitr. Path. 145, 336–349 (1972).

Palade, G. E.: A small particulate component of the cytoplasm. In: Frontiers in cytology. New Haven: Yale Univ. Press 1958.

Palay, S. L., Karlin, L. J.: An electron microscopic study of the intestinal villus. II. The pathway of fat absorption. J. biophys. biochem. Cytol. 5, 373–384 (1959).

Papermaster, B. W., Condie, R. M., Finstad, J., Good, R. A.: Evolution of the immune response. I. The phylogenetic development of adaptive immunologic responsiveness in vertebrates. J. exp. Med. 119, 105–130 (1964).

Parker, J. W., Wakasa, H., Lukes, R. J.: The morphologic and cytochemical demonstration of lysosomes in lymphocytes with Phytohaemagglutinin by electron microscopy. Lab. Invest. 14, 1736–1743 (1965).

Patzelt, V.: Der Darm. In: Handbuch der mikroskopischen Anatomie des Menschen, Bd. V/3. Berlin: Springer 1936.

PERLMANN, P., HAMMARSTRÖM, S., LAGERCRANTZ, R., CAMPBELL, D.: Autoantibodies to colon in rats and human ulcerative colitis: Crossreactivity with escherichia coli o14 antigen. Proc. Soc. exp. Biol. (N.Y.) **125**, 975–980 (1967).

PERLMANN, P., HOLM, G.: (1969) cited by FISCHER, H., RÜDE, E., SELLIN, D. Naturwissenschaften **57**, 507–513 (1970).

PFEIFFER, C. J., WEIBEL, J.: The antral clear cell — a new cell type discovered in the pyloric-antral mucosa of the ferret. J. Ultrastruct. Res. **29**, 550–562 (1969).

POLITOFF, A. L., SOCOLAR, S. J., LOEWENSTEIN, W. R.: Permeability of a cell membrane junction. Dependence on energy metabolism. J. gen. Physiol. **53**, 498–515 (1969).

RAFF, M. C., STERNBERG, M., TAYLOR, R. B.: Immunoglobulin determinants on the surface of mouse lymphoid cells. Nature (Lond.) **225**, 553–554 (1970).

RINDFLEISCH, E.: Über die Entstehung des Eiters auf Schleimhäuten. Virchows Arch. path. Anat. **21**, 486–505 (1861).

ROGERS, A. I.: Immunoglobulins and the gastrointestinal tract. Postgrad. Med. **48**, 75–82 (1970).

ROOS, B.: Makrophagen: Herkunft, Entwicklung und Funktion. In: Handbuch der allgemeinen Pathologie, Bd. VII/3. Berlin-Heidelberg-New York: Springer 1970.

RUBIN, C. E., BRANDBORG, L. L., FLICK, A. L., MacDONALD, W. C., PARKINS, R. A., PARMENTIER, CH., PHELPS, M., SRIBHIBHADH, S., TRIER, J. S.: Biopsy studies on the pathogenesis of coeliac sprue. In: Intestinal biopsy. London: Ciba Foundation, Study Group No 14 1962.

RUBIN, W.: Celiac disease. Amer. J. clin. Nutr. **24**, 91–111 (1971).

RUBIN, W., FAUCI, A. S., SLEISINGER, M. H., JEFFRIES, G. H.: Immunofluorescent studies in adult celiac disease. J. clin. Invest. **44**, 475–485 (1965).

SAITO, T., HONMA, T., SATO, T., FUJIOKA, Y.: Auto-immune mechanisms as a probable aetiology of Behcet's syndrome, an electron microscopic study of the oral mucosa., Virchows Arch. Abt. A **353**, 261–272 (1971).

SATAKE, K.: Über die Lymphozyten in der Darmschleimhaut. Trans. jap. path. Soc. **14**, 81–82 (1924).

SATAKE, K.: Experimentelle Beiträge zur Theorie der enteralen Funktion der Lymphozyten. Sci. Rep. Gov. Inst. inf. Dis. Tokyo **13**, 121–158 (1924b).

SCHÄFER, E. A.: Cited by PATZELT, V.: Der Darm. In: Handbuch der mikroskopischen Anatomie des Menschen, Bd. V/3. Berlin: Springer 1936.

SCHAFFER, J.: Beiträge zur Histologie menschlicher Organe. I. Duodenum. II. Dünndarm. III. Mastdarm. S.-B. Akad. Wiss. Wien, math.-nat. Kl. III **100**, 440–481 (1891).

SCHAFFER, J.: Victor von Ebner zum Gedächtnis. Anat. Anz. **64**, 1–50 (1927).

SCHAUER, A., GERSTER, H.: Die Mastzelle bei akuten Überempfindlichkeitsreaktionen. In: Handbuch der allgemeinen Pathologie, Bd. VII/3. Berlin-Heidelberg-New York: Springer 1970.

SCHOFIELD, G. C.: Columnar cells with secretory granules in the large intestine of the macaque (Cynamolgus irus). J. Anat. (Lond.) **106**, 1–14 (1970).

SHIELDS, J. W., TOUCHON, R. C., DICKSON, D. R.: Quantitative studies on small lymphocyte disposition in epithelial cells. Amer. J. Path. **54**, 129–145 (1969).

SHORTER, R. G., CARDOZA, M., SPENCER, R. J., HUIZENGA, K. A.: Further studies of in vitro cytotoxicity of lymphocytes from patients with ulcerative and granulomatous colitis for allogenic colonic epithelial cells, including the effects of colectomy. Gastroenterology **56**, 304–309 (1969).

SHORTER, R. G., SPENCER, R. J., HUIZENGA, K. A., HALLENBECK, G. A.: Inhibition of in vitro cytotoxicity of lymphocytes from patients with ulcerative colitis and granulomatous colitis for allogenic colonic epithelial cells using horse antihuman thymus serum. Gastroenterology **54**, 227–231 (1968).

SIEKEVITZ, P.: The cytological basis of protein synthesis. Exp. Cell Ses., Suppl. **7**,90–110 (1959).

SIEKEVITZ, P.: Ribonucleoprotein particles as templates for protein synthesis. In: Protein biosynthesis. New York: Academic Press, Inc. 1961.

SILVA, D. G.: The ultrastructure of crystal-containing cells in the colonic epithelium of mice. J. Ultrastruct. Res. **18**, 127–141 (1967).

SIRTORI, C.: Blastic transformation in leucocyte cultures. Lancet **1967I**, 215.

SLANEY, G.: Intestinal response to immunologic insult. Amer. Surg. **115**, 457–464 (1968).

SMITHIES, O.: Cited by FISCHER, H., RÜDE, E., SELLIN, D.: Membranaspekte der Immunologie. Naturwissenschaften 57, 507–513 (1970).

SØLTOFT, J.: Immunoglobulin-containing cells in normal jejunal mucosa and in ulcerative colitis and regional enteritis. Scand. J. Gastroent. 4, 353–360 (1969).

SØLTOFT, J.: Immunoglobulin-containing cells in nontropical sprue. Clin. exp. Immunol. 6, 413–420 (1970).

SOUTH, M. A., COOPER, M. D., WOLLHEIM, F. A., GOOD, R. A.: The IgA system. II. The clinical significance of IgA deficiency: Studies in patients with agammaglobulinemia and ataxiatelangiectasia. Amer. J. Med. 44, 168–178 (1968).

SOUTH, M. A., WARWICK, W. J., WOLLHEIM, F. A., GOOD, R. A.: The IgA system. III. IgA levels in the serum and saliva of pediatric patients — evidence for a local immunological system. J. Pediat. 71, 645–653 (1967).

STENQUIST, H.: Die „Zellwanderung" durch das Darmepithel. Anat. Anz. 78, 68–79 (1934).

STEVENS, B. J., SWIFT, H.: RNA transport from nucleus to cytoplasm in Chironomus salivary glands. J. Cell Biol. 31, 55–77 (1966).

STILLMAN, A., ZAMCHECK, N.: Recent advances in immunologic diagnosis of digestive tract cancer. Amer. J. dig. Dis. 15, 1003–1018 (1970).

STOECKENIUS, W.: Zur Feinstruktur der Granula menschlicher Gewebsmastzellen. Exp. Cell Res. 11, 656–658 (1956).

STÖHR, PH.: Über die peripheren Lymphdrüsen. S.-B. phys. med. Ges. Würzb. 86–94 (1883).

STÖHR, PH.: Über die Lymphknötchen des Darmes. Arch. mikr. Anat. 33, 255–283 (1889).

STÖHR, PH.: Verdauungs-Apparat. Ergebn. Anat. Entwickl.-Gesch. 1, 173–196 (1891/92).

TAKEUCHI, A., JERVIS, H. R., SPRINZ, H.: The globule leucocyte in the intestinal mucosa of the cat. A histochemical, light and electron microscopic study. Anat. Rec. 164, 79–99 (1969).

TANAKA, Y., EPSTEIN, L. B., BRECHER, G., STOHLMAN, F., JR.: Transformation of lymphocytes in cultures of human peripheral blood. Blood 22, 614–629 (1963).

THAYER, W. R., BROWN, M., SANGREE, M. H., KATZ, J., HERSH, T.: Escherichia coli 014 and colon hemagglutinating antibodies in inflammatory bowel disease. Gastroenterology 57, 311–318 (1969).

THIÉRY, J. P.: Etude au microscope électronique de la maturation et de l'excretion des granules des mastocytes. J. Micr. 2, 549–556 (1963).

TÖRÖ, E.: Bedeutung und Entstehung der Zellgranula in der Darmresorption. Z. Anat. Entwickl.-Gesch. 94, 1–38 (1931).

TOMASI, T. B.: Human immunoglobulin. A. New Engl. J. Med. 279, 1327–1330 (1968).

TOMASI, T. B.: Structure and function of mucosal antibodies. Ann. Rev. Med. 21, 281–298 (1970).

TOMASI, T. B., BIENENSTOCK, J.: Secretory immunoglobulins. Advanc. Immunol. 9, 1–96 (1968).

TONER, P. G.: The fine structure of the globule leucocyte in the fowl intestine. Acta anat. (Basel) 61, 321–330 (1965).

TONER, P. G.: Cytology intestinel epithelial cells. Int. Rec. Cytol. 24, 233–343 (1968).

TONER, P. G., CARR, K. E., WYBURN, G. M.: The digestive system-an ultrastructural atlas and review. London: Butterworths 1971.

TONER, P. G., FERGUSON, A.: Intraepithelial cells in the human intestinal mucosa. J. Ultrastruct. Res. 34, 329—344 (1971).

TOUJAS, L., GUELFI, J.: Sur l'ultrastructure de la glande thyroide humaine. Z. Zellforsch. 94, 118–128 (1969).

TROWELL, O. A.: The lymphocyte. Int. Rev. Cytol. 7, 235–293 (1958).

UNANUE, E. R., ASKONAS, B. A.: Persistence of immunogenicity of antigen after uptake by macrophages. J. exp. Med. 127, 915–926 (1968).

UNANUE, E. R., ASKONAS, B. A., ALLISON, A. C.: A role of macrophages in the stimulation of immune response by adjuvants. J. Immunol. 103, 71–78 (1969).

VISAKORPI, J. K., IMMONEN, P.: Intolerance to cow's milk and wheat gluten in the primary malabsorption syndrome in infancy. Acta paediat. scand. 56, 49–56 (1967).

VOGT, W., HAUSSMANN, P., BOHLE, A.: Über lympho-epitheliale Beziehungen in menschlichen Nierentransplantaten. Klin. Wschr. 48, 1327–1330 (1970).

WAELE, H. DE: Recherches sur le rôle des globules blancs dans l'absorption chez les vertébrés. Livre jubil. Ch. v. Bambeke. Bruxelles 1899.

WAKSMAN, B. H.: A comparative histopathological study of delayed hypersensitive reactions. In: Cellular aspects of immunity. Ciba Foundation Symposium. Boston: Little, Brown & Co. 1960.

WAKSMAN, B. H.: The pattern of rejection in rat skin homografts, and its relationship to the vascular network. Lab. Invest. 12, 46–57 (1963).

WAKSMAN, B. H.: The local reaction of cellular hypersensitivity. Ann. N.Y. Acad. Sci. 116, 1045–1051 (1964).

WALKE, A.: Über lympho-epitheliale Beziehungen bei Proctocolitis ulcerosa und Morbus Crohn. Morphologische und statistische Untersuchungen. Med. Diss., Hamburg 1972.

WALL, A. J., DOUGLAS, A. P., BOOTH, C. C., PEARSE, A. G. E.: Response of the jejunal mucosa in adult coeliac disease to oral prednisolone. Gut 11, 7–14 (1970).

WATNEY, H.: The minute anatomy of the alimentary canal. Phil. Trans. Roy. Soc. Lond. 166, 451–488 (1877).

WATSON, D. W.: The lymphocyte and ulcerative colitis. Gastroenterology 56, 385–386 (1969).

WATSON, D. W.: Immune response and the gut. Gastroenterology 56, 944–965 (1969).

WATSON, D. W., BOLT, R. J.: Immune mechanism and ulcerative colitis. In: Progress in gastroenterology, vol. I. New York: Grune and Stratton 1968.

WATSON, D. W., QUIGLEY, A., BOLT, R. J.: Effect of lymphocytes from patients with ulcerative colitis on human adult colon epithelial cells. Gastroenterology 51, 985–993 (1966).

WATSON, M. L.: Further observations on the nuclear envelope of the animal cell. J. biophys. biochem. Cytol. 6, 147–156 (1959).

WATZKA, M.: Epithel und Lymphozyt. Verh. anat. Ges. (Jena) 41, 150–158 (1932).

WEBER, E. H.: Über den Mechanismus der Einsaugung des Speisesaftes beim Menschen und bei einigen Tieren. Arch. Anat. Physiol. u. wiss. Med. 1847, 400–402.

WEILL, P.: Über die leukocytären Elemente der Darmschleimhaut der Säugetiere. Arch. mikr. Anat. 93, 1–81 (1920).

WEINSTEIN, R. S.: Current concepts. The structure of cell membranes. New Engl. J. Med. 281, 86-89 (1969).

WEINSTEIN, R. S., SOMEDA, K.: Cited by FISCHER, H., RÜDE, E., SELLIN, D., Naturwissenschaften 57, 507–513 (1970).

WEINSTOCK, A., ALBRIGHT, J. T.: The fine structure of mast cells in normal human gingiva. J. Ultrastruct. Res. 17, 245–256 (1967).

WEITZ, H.: Ultrastrukturelle Untersuchungen an den Paneth-Zellen des Rattendünndarms unter zinkarmer Diät und Äthionineinwirkung. Diss. Med., Hamburg 1972.

WIENER, J.: Ultrastructural aspects of delayed hypersensitivity. Curr. Top. Pathol. 52, 143–208 (1970).

WIENER, J., SPIRO, D., RUSSELL, P. S.: Electron microscope studies of the homograft reaction. In: Proc. Fifth International Congress for Electron Microscopy, vol. II. New York: Academic Press, Inc. 1962.

WIENER, J., SPIRO, D., RUSSELL, P. S.: An electron microscopic study of the homograft reaction. Amer. J. Path. 44, 319–347 (1964).

WOLF-HEIDEGGER, G.: Zur Frage der Lymphozytenwanderung durch das Darmepithel. Z. mikr. anat. Forsch. 45, 90–103 (1939).

YOFFREY, J. M.: The fourth circulation. In: The lymphocyte in immunology and haemopoiesis. London: Arnold 1967.

ZIETZSCHMANN, O.: Über die acidophilen Leukocyten (Körnerzellen) des Pferdes. Internat. Mschr. Anat. Physiol. 22, 1–89 (1905).

Multiple Deep Fungus Infections:

Personal Observations and a Critical Review of the World Literature*

K. Salfelder, M. Mendelovici, and J. Schwarz

With 10 Figures

Contents

A. Introduction

Interest in the deep mycoses has been on the increase, stimulated in part by improved diagnostic methods and in part by a higher incidence in discovery. Additional factors in this increased interest have been wider geographic

* This work was supported in part by the CONICIT (Consejo Nacional de Investigaciones Científicas y Tecnológicas), Caracas and the Consejo de Desarrollo Científico y Humanístico de la ULA, Mérida/Venezuela.

recognition, contributing to an internationality far beyond the so-called endemic areas, and actual spread of the involved organisms stimulated by today's international *Reise-Kultur*.

A major difficulty in such a study has been lack of standardization. Terminology and taxonomy not only vary greatly between nations but even within nations. The taxonomy of fungi and similar lower organisms is in a state of flux, as evidenced by the 1970 edition of *Medical Mycology* [27]. Emmons [27] shares the currently widespread view, that fungi should be considered as separate kingdom (Whittaker [114]).

Obviously, this revolutionary approach makes for considerable confusion, particularly since there are good reasons to separate Actinomycetaceae and Nocardia-Species from fungi altogether. The reasons for considering the actinomycetaceae as bacteria relate to the chemical composition of the cell wall (presence of muramic and diaminopimelic acid; absence of chitin, a typical constituent of the cell wall of molds and yeasts); sensitivity to antibacterial drugs like penicillins and tetracyclines; lack of nuclear membrane; fragmentation into bacillary forms (Whittaker [114]). The result is a certain inconsistency, as in the exclusion of *Pneumocystis carinii* from the fungus group and including *Pneumocystis* in the phylum Protista.

The nomenclature of mycoses caused by certain coenocytic fungi is open to discussion. The original term, mucormycosis, was replaced by phycomycosis, which we use in this paper. Clark [20] has recently suggested that mucormycosis would be valid for diseases caused by the order Mucorales. All diseases including subcutaneous phycomycosis, Clark would propose to call entomophthoromycosis, a term, which appears to be somewhat hard to swallow and to pronounce, even if good theoretical reasons can be brought forward to call diseases caused by the order Entomophthorales by their proper name.

In this study, "dissemination" means involvement of two or more non-contiguous visceral organs. In table 1, involvement of two organs was specified. "Localised", refers to the involvement of one organ or one system (lung and regional lymph nodes, for example). "Active" means more or less extensive and recent tissue lesions with potentiality of spread. "Residual" indicates circumscribed, nonactive, burned-out foci without further potentiality for dissemination. Cases with confirmation of two fungus species in one lesion were also considered as multiple mycoses.

Further, "popular" acceptance of actinomycosis, nocardiosis, and pneumocystosis among the common systemic fungus infections has led us to include these conditions in our study, despite their not being true mycoses.

B. Method

All reports of cases involving more than one mycosis were collected and reviewed, so far as these were available in the world literature. Distinction was made between active cases of mycosis *in vivo* and the findings of several fungi at necropsy, as in the reports of SICHERT and MAHNKE [88], MAHNKE *et al.* [55], VANBREUSEGHEM [108], and ALKIEWICZ *et al.* [3].

Table 1 lists the main data of 197 cases. Thirteen cases are included which have not yet been published: 6 from Japan with data kindly provided by M. OKUDAIRA* (138–143), 5 from CINCINNATI, U.S.A. (147, 187–190) and 2 from MÉRIDA, Venezuela (182, 184). The cases in Table 1 are listed in order of the year of publication. One case reported as early as 1939 by ALMEIDA and LACAZ, mentioned by BOPP and LIMA [13], was not included (see chapter 20).

From 1947–1952, only one case per year was reported; until 1961, a few cases per year. The bulk of the casuistic reports appear from 1962 on, with 31 cases in 1967 alone (Table 2).

Cases were reported from only 9 countries. In order of frequency, USA 122; Japan 27; Great Britain 22; Venezuela 15; Colombia 4; Brazil 3; Germany 2; Costa Rica 1; Switzerland 1. More than two thirds of all cases were from North, Central, and South America. From Europe, the largest number were from Great Britain, and from Asia, the only cases, were from Japan. No cases could be found reported, from Africa, Australia, Russia, or China.

The majority of cases were collected and described by a few authors: ZIMMERMAN and RAPPAPORT [120], BRANDSBERG *et al.* [14], HUTTER and COLLINS [43], GRUHN and SANSON [39], PREISLER *et al.* [71], from the USA; SYMMERS [96–100] from Great Britain; MIYAKE and OKUDAIRA [60] from Japan. This points only to the fact that the subject was of special interest to these authors and should not be interpreted to mean that multiple fungus infections occur only in these nine countries; in other countries, apparently, they were simply not published or publications were not available.

Cytology: *H. capsulatum*, in clusters and uniform in size, is unique in appearance in tissue. *Blastomyces dermatitidis*, with its thick wall, broad-based single bud, and multiple nuclei, can be identified also in tissues. *P. brasiliensis*, if found with multiple buds, is likewise acceptable by morphology alone.

Cryptococcus neoformans almost always shows the characteristic mucine-positive capsules, and the endospores containing sporangia of *Coccidioides immitis*, if present, are also characteristic in histologic sections and smears. The same applies to Candida species showing yeast cells and pseudohyphae side by side.

On the other hand, we consider it unwise to rely upon morphology alone in the diagnosis of sporotrichosis and aspergillosis. Unless clear-cut vesicles with sterigmata are demonstrated in aspergillosis we do not make this diagnosis on our own material based on the simple presence of branching septate hyphae, whether or not the hyphae grow unidirectionally, as the chances of error are high. Phycomyces generally can be recognized from the width of the hyphae and the absence of septa; however, at least two precautions should be mentioned: (1), many young hyphae from a variety of fungi lack septa and therefore the age of development of fungal infection must be considered, and (2),

---

* We are especially grateful to Dr. M. OKUDAIRA, Tokyo, who gave us detailed data for most of the Japanese cases.

Table 1. Details

Nr.	Year	Author	Country	Age, sex	Race occupat. origin	A	Mycoses
1	1947	Mider *et al.* [59]	U.S.A.	12, ♂	negro Virginia	+	Histopl. dissemin. Cryptoc. dissemin.
2	1948	Spicer *et al.* [92]	U.S.A.	8, ♂	white	+	Cryptoc. dissemin. Candid. dissemin.
3	1950	Mosberg and Arnold [62]	U.S.A.	18, ♂	white	+	Cryptoc. CNS Candid. dissemin. (C. alb.)
4	1951	Rodger *et al.* [76]	U.S.A.	38, ♂	white	+	Histopl. dissemin. Cryptoc. skin.
5	1952	Abbott *et al.* [1]	Great Brit.	51, ♀		+	Candid. lung (C. alb.) Aspergill. lung (A. fum.)
6	1953	Layton *et al.* [49]	U.S.A.	46, ♂	Iowa	+	Histopl. dissemin. Blastom. dissemin.
7	1953	Leopold [52]	U.S.A.	37, ♀			Cryptoc. bone Candid. lung
8	1953	Rankin [73]	U.S.A.	45, ♂		+	Asperg. dissemin. Candid. dissemin.
9	1954	Vivian *et al.* [109]	U.S.A.	30, ♂			Histopl. lung. Cryptoc. (*)
10	1954	Zimmerman and Rappaport [120]	U.S.A.	59, ♂	negro	+	Cryptoc. dissemin. Coccid. (*)
11	1954	Zimmerman and Rappaport [120]	U.S.A.	46, ♂		+	Histopl. adrenal Cryptoc. CNS
12	1954	Zimmerman and Rappaport [120]	U.S.A.	35, ♂	white	+	Histopl. (*) Cryptoc. dissemin.
13	1954	Zimmerman and Rappaport [120] (Cross and Binford, 1962) [22]	U.S.A.	25, ♂	white	+	Cryptoc. dissemin. Nocardiosis lung
14	1955	Levy and Cohen [53]	U.S.A.	24, ♀	white	+	Asperg. dissemin. Candid. dissemin.
15	1956	Walz *et al.* [111]	U.S.A.	4, ♂	white	+	Cryptoc. dissemin. Candid. dissemin. (no Aut. of head)
16	1956	Straub and Schwarz [94]	U.S.A.	81, ♂	white Arizona Indiana	+	Histopl. lung (primary complex) Coccid. residual

A = autopsy performed,   H = post-mortem histology,   Cam = ante-mortem culture, oculation into animals,   FAT = fluorescent antibody technic,   antib = antibiotics, (x) = case not published,   (*) = organs involved not mentioned,   (+) = degree of paraon multiple mycoses

| Diagns. methods | | | | | | | Associated disease(s) | Treatment |
H	B	Cam	Cpm	Ed	Im	In		
+			+	+				
+			+					
+		+	+					irrad., iodides, autovaccin, gentian violet i.V., antib.
+		+	+			+		
+		+				+		irrad., antib., fevertherapy kayquinone
+			+					
+	+	+	+				Hodgkin, Tub. diss.	orchidectomy for Tub., Pentamidine, Stibanose
	+							
		+	+				bronchopneu-monia	antib.
+			+					
+			+				duodenal and esophag. ulcer	
+			+					
		+				+		sulf., iodides, autovaccin, antib
		+			+			
+							abscess of thigh agranulocytosis	antib.
+								
		+			+		anemia	
		+						
+							hepatic cirrhosis	
+							hypertension, uremia	
+								
+								
+							Hodgkin, Tub.	
+	+							
+		+		+			chron. myelog. leukemia	urethane, irrad. antib.
+								
+		+	+				anemia, thrombo-cytopenia, terminal staphylo septicemia	ster. antib.
+		+	+					
+			+				lipoid nephrosis	ster. antib. ACTH
+		+	+					
+							cardiac	
+								

Cpm = post-mortem-culture,   Ed = direct examination,   Im = immunology,   In = in-
Irrad = irradiation,   ster = steroids,   tub = tuberculosis,   cytost = cytostatics.
sitism of P. carinii, ∅ = negative.

Table 1

Nr.	Year	Author	Country	Age, sex	Race occupat. origin	A	Mycoses
17	1956	Straub and Schwarz [94]	U.S.A.	54, ♂	white Illinois	+	Histopl. lung. residual Coccid. lung, residual
18	1956	Straub and Schwarz [94]	U.S.A.	60, ♂	white Italian Arizona	+	Histopl. lung, residual Coccid. lung, residual
19	1957	Bopp y Lima [13]	Brasil	46, ♂	white farmer		Chromom. foot, leg Sporotr. finger Paracocci lung
20	1957	Torack [102]	U.S.A.	57, ♀	white	+	Aspergill. lung Candid. upper digestive tract
21	1957	Torack [102]	U.S.A.	65, ♂	white	+	Aspergill. lung Candid. stomach
22	1957	Torack [102]	U.S.A.	45, ♂	white	+	Aspergill. lung. Candid. stomach
23	1959	Finegold et al. [30]	U.S.A.	62, ♂	white	+	Aspergill. lung Candid. lung esoph.
24	1959	Hutter [42]	U.S.A.	62, ♂	white	+	Phycom. lung, spleen Candid. esoph. (no Auto. of head)
25	1959	Hutter [42]	U.S.A.	8, ♂		+	Phycom. dissemin. (Mucor sp.) Candid. upp. digest tract
26	1959	Hutter [42]	U.S.A.	8, ♂	white	+	Phycom. dissemin. Candid. digest. tract
27	1959	Winslow and Hathaway [117] (Symmers, 1960) [97]	U.S.A.	39, ♂		+	Cryptoc. dissemin. Histopl. lung residual Pneum. car. (+ + +)
28	1960	Frenkel [33]	U.S.A.	43, ♂	white	+	Histopl. dissem. resid. adren, spl. Cryptoc. lung
29	1960	Gowing and Hamlin [38]	U.S.A.	41, ♀		+	Aspergill. lung Candid. upp. dig. tr
30	1960	Procknow and Loewen [72]	U.S.A.	28, ♂	white Illinois		Histopl. lung, cured Aspergill. lung (fung. ball)
31	1960	Symmers [97]	Great Brit.	47, ♂		+	Cryptoc. lung Pneum. car. (+ +) (limited Aut.)

(Continued)

Diagns. methods							Associated disease(s)	Treatment
H	B	Cam	Cpm	Ed	Im	In		
+							subarrachnoid	
+							hemorrhagia	
+							pyelonephritis	
+								
+				+				
		+						
				+		+		
+							anaplastic carcinoma	irrad. antib.
+		+					breast (mastectomy), post-radiation leuko-penia	ster.
+							anaplastic carcinoma	irrad. antib.
+							bladder (ureterostomy, colostomy)	
+							Hodgkin, pancyto-penia	antib. ster. ACTH
+								
+							epidermoid carcinoma hypoplastic anemia and leukopenia staphylo pneumonia	antib. ster.
+								
+							acute myelogenous leukemia	antib, ster.
+								
+			+				lymphosarcoma, post-radiation fibrosis of kidneys	irrad, ster, cytostatics Mycostatin
+								
+							acute leukemia ster. induced hyperglycemia	antib. ster cytost.
+								
+							chronic lymphat. leukemia	antib, irrad, ster Au*
+								
+								
		+	+				bronchopneumonia	stilbamidina, ster
+			+					
+								
+							Hodgkin (block dissection of lymph nodes) staphylo abscess lung	irrad, antib, ster
+								
				+				resection lung
	+	+						
+	+						microangiopathy general cytomeg. vir. incl., agenesis of spleen	antib, ster.
+								

Table 1

Nr.	Year	Author	Country	Age, sex	Race occupat. origin	A	Mycoses
32	1961	Angulo O. *et al.* [5]	Vene-zuela	47, ♂		+	Cryptoc. lung, CNS Paracocci lung, mucosa buccal
33	1961	Schwarz *et al.* [86]	U.S.A.	45, ♂	white Ohio	+	Histopl. lung Aspergill. lung (fung ball)
34	1961	Schwarz *et al.* [86]	U.S.A.	47, ♂	white Ohio		Histopl. lung Aspergill. lung (fung. ball)
35	1961	Schwarz *et al.* [86]	U.S.A.	49, ♂	white Ohio	+	Histopl. lung Aspergill. lung (fung. ball)
36	1961	Schwarz *et al.* [86]	U.S.A.	70, ♂	white Ohio		Histopl. lung Aspergill. lung (fung. ball, diagn. radiol.)
37	1961	Sidransky and Pearl [89]	U.S.A.	29, ♀	white	+	Aspergill. lung (A. flavus) Candid. dissemin.
38	1961	Utz *et al.* [105]	U.S.A.	66, ♂	white farmer		Histopl. lung Aspergill. lung
39	1961	Utz *et al.* [105]	U.S.A.	61, ♂	white farmer		Cryptoc. CNS Mycetoma ankle (Mad. grisea)
40	1962	Allison *et al.* [4]	U.S.A.	43, ♂	white farmer Missis-sippi		Histopl. lung, lar. Blastom. lung
41	1962	Baker [6]	U.S.A.	50, ♂	black	+	Phycom. dissemin. (Mucor sp.) Aspergill. lung Candid. esoph.
42	1962	Baker [6]	U.S.A.	70, ♂		+	Phycom. lung (Mucor sp.) Aspergill. brain
43	1962	Saltzman *et al.* [82] (Cross and Binford, 1962) [22]	U.S.A.	32, ♂	white	+	Nocard. lung (N. ast) Aspergill. myocard.
44	1962	Cross and Binford [22]	U.S.A.	59, ♂	white	+	Nocard. lung Aspergill. lung
45	1962	Furcolow [34] (Morris *et al.*, 1964) [61]	U.S.A.	66, ♂	white Kansas	+	Histopl dissemin. Cryptoc. dissemin. Candid. dissemin.
46	1962	Hendry and Patrick [40]	U.S.A.	6, ♀	white	+	Candid. lung P. carinii (+)

(Continued)

| Diagns. methods | | | | | | | Associated disease(s) | Treatment |
H	B	Cam	Cpm	Ed	Im	In		
+			+				Tub. lung andly node	
+	+	+	+				anemia, intestin.	
							parasitosis	
+		+					psychotic,	
+							cachexia	
					+		cirrhosis, duodenal	Amphot. B, 5 mo
	+	+					ulcer chron. chole-	
							cyst. bronchitis	
+					+		chronic bronchitis	
+								
		+			+			Amph. B, 870 mg
								Amph. B, 2,500 mg
+			+				agranulocytosis	antib, ster.
							septicemia with	
+		+	+				Staph. aur. and Aero-	
							bact. aerog.	
	+	+			+			antib, X5079C
	+							
		+						stilbam, Amphot. B
	+	+						X5079 C
	+	+		+	+		arthritis	antib, inj, of Au,
	+	+			+	+		ster (3y), Amph. B
								(tot. 6 g)
+			+				chronic lymphoc.	
+			+				leukemia	
+								
+			+				acute myeloblastic	splenectomy
							leukemia	irrad, antib, ster
+								cytost.
+			+				Cushing	subtotal adrenalectomy,
+								antib, ster
+							ulcerat. colitis	ster, antib.
+								
+		+	+		FAT			Amph. B: 350 mg, I.V.
+		+						and 12,5 mg. I th.
+					FAT			Amph. B: 10 mg. I.V.
+							monocytic leukemia	antib, ster,
+								cytotox.

9*

Table 1

Nr.	Year	Author	Country	Age, sex	Race occupat. origin	A	Mycoses
47	1962	Hendry and Patrick [40]	U.S.A.	10, ♂	white	+	Candid. dissemin. P. carinii (+)
48	1962	Hendry and Patrick [40]	U.S.A.	20, ♂	white	+	Candid. lung P. carinii (+++)
49	1962	Hendry and Patrick [40]	U.S.A.	52, ♀	colored	+	Cryptoc. dissemin. Nocard. dissemin. P. carinii
50–54	1962	Hutter and Collins [43]	U.S.A.				Candidosis (*) Aspergillosis (*)
55	1962	Hutter and Collins [43]	U.S.A.				Candidosis (*) Aspergillosis (*) Geotrichosis (*)
56–58	1962	Hutter and Collins [43]	U.S.A.				Geotrichosis (*) Candidosis (*)
59–60	1962	Hutter and Collins [43]	U.S.A.				Cryptococ. (*) Candidosis (*)
61	1962	Hutter and Collins [43]	U.S.A.				Cryptoc. (*) Phycom. (*) Candidosis (*)
62	1962	Hutter and Collins [43]	U.S.A.				Phycom. (*) Geotrich. (*)
63	1962	Hutter and Collins [43]	U.S.A.				Candidosis (*) Nocardiosis (*)
64	1962	Straatsma et al. [93]	U.S.A.	65, ♀		+	Cryptoc. dissemin. Phycom. brain
65	1962	Utz [106]	U.S.A.				Actinom. cervical Coccid. lung
66	1963	Gilbert et al. [37]	U.S.A.	42, ♀	white	+	Aspergill. lung P. carinii (+++)
67	1963	Gruhn and Sanson [39]	U.S.A.	29, ♀		+	Nocard. lung Candid. esoph. intest.
68	1963	Gruhn and Sanson [39]	U.S.A.	67, ♀		+	Aspergill. lung Candid. stomach
69	1963	Gruhn and Sanson [39]	U.S.A.	73, ♀		+	Aspergill. lung Candid. heart, kidney
70	1963	Gruhn and Sanson [39]	U.S.A.	68, ♀		+	Aspergill. dissemin. Candid. dissemin.
71	1963	Gruhn and Sanson [39]	U.S.A.	50, ♀		+	Phycom. lung, brain Aspergill. lung
72	1963	Gruhn and Sanson [39]	U.S.A.	59, ♀		+	Aspergill. lung Candid. esoph.

(Continued)

Diagns. methods							Associated disease(s)	Treatment
H	B	Cam	Cpm	Ed	Im	In		
+							aplastic anemia	antib, ster.
+							FANCONI's syndr.	
							bacter. pneumonia	
+			+				lymphoblastic	antib, ster,
+							leukemia, staphylo	cytost.
							lung	
+							multiple myeloma	antib, cytotox.
+								
+								
							cancer	
			+				cancer	
			+					
			+					
			+				cancer	
			+					
							cancer	
							cancer	
							cancer	
							cancer	
+							renal insuff.	
+								
+		+					chron. lymphoc.	irrad, antib, ster
+							leukemia	cytost.
+							acute stem cell	ster, antib
+							leukemia	cytost.
+							acute granuloc.	antib, ster
+							leukemia	
+							acute lymphoc.	ster, antib.
+		+					leukemia	
+							chron. granuloc.	antib, ster,
+							leukemia	cytostat.
							staphylococcemia	
+							lymphosarcoma	antib, ster.
+							chron. lymphoc.	
							leukemia	
+							chron. lymphoc.	antib, ster,
+							leukemia	cytost.

Table 1

Nr.	Year	Author	Country	Age, sex	Race occupat. origin	A	Mycoses
73	1963	La Touche et al. [48]	Great Brit.	58, ♀		+	Candid. nasal pasages (C. alb.) Phycom. rhinocerebr. (Rhizop. oryzae)
74	1963	Saenz J. y Morera [78]	Costa Rica	54, ♂	white		Paracocc. lung, oral cavity Chromomyc. legs
75	1963	Straub et al. [95]	U.S.A.			+	Histo resid. lung Cocci resid. lung
76	1963	Wahner et al. [110]	U.S.A.	2, ♂	farmer's son	+	Asperg. lung, pericard, ulcer Penicill. lung
77	1964	Brandsberg et al. [14]	U.S.A.	74, ♂	Kentucky		Histopl. lung Blastom. lung
78	1964	Brandsberg et al. [14]	U.S.A.	47, ♂	farmer Texas		Histopl. lung Blastom. lung
79	1964	Brandsberg et al. [14]	U.S.A.	54, ♂	merchant seaman		Histopl. lung Blastom. lung, skin
80	1964	Brandsberg et al. [14]	U.S.A.	69, ♂	farmer Kentucky		Histopl. lung Blastom. lung
81	1964	Brandsberg et al. [14]	U.S.A.	47, ♂	machinist Missouri		Histopl. lung Blastom. lung
82	1964	Hill et al. [41]	U.S.A.	25, ♂		+	Aspergill. dissem. (Asp. fumig.) Candid. dissem. (Cand. alb.)
83	1964	Hill et al. [41]	U.S.A.	30, ♂		+	Nocard. dissem. (N. ast.) Candid. lung (Cand. alb.)
84	1964	Magaldi et al. [54]	Brasil	18, ♀	colored		Cryptoc. lung Candid. lung
85	1964	Magaldi et al. [54]	Brasil	34, ♀	japanese	+	Cryptoc. dissemin. Candid. lung
86	1965	Esterly and Warner [28]	U.S.A.	9, ♂	caucasian	+	Candid. lung Penicill. lung P. carinii (+++)
87	1965	Esterly and Warner [28]	U.S.A.	54, ♀	caucasian	+	Candid. lung P. carinii (+)
88	1965	Esterly and Warner [28]	U.S.A.	30, ♀	caucasian	+	Aspergill. lung (A. fum.) P. carinii (+++)
89	1965	Esterly and Warner [28]	U.S.A.	81, ♂	caucasian	+	Aspergill. lung (A. fum.) P. carinii (++++)

(Continued)

Diagns. methods							Associated disease(s)	Treatment
H	B	Cam	Cpm	Ed	Im	In		
∅		+					Diabetes	Nystatine local
+	+	+						
	+	+		+			Tub. anemia	
	+						Intest. parasites	
+								
+								
+	+	+	+				strepto-septicem.	KI
∅	+	+						
		+			+			
		+			+			
		+			+		accidental para-plegia	
		+						
	+	+			+ FAT		tub. lung	
	+	+			FAT			
		+			+			
	+	+			+ FAT			
		+						
		+			+			
+			+				renal transplant	ster, cytost, azathioprin
+			+					
+			+				renal transplant	ster, cytost, azathioprin
+			+				cytomeg. vir.	
			∅	+		+	intest. parasites	
	+	+						
+		+		+			Toxoplasmosis	
		+		+			amibiasis	
			+				stem cell leukemia	antib, ster, cytost.
+								
			+					
+							Hodgkin	irrad. antib. ster cytost.
			+				stem cell leuk	ster, antib, cytost.
+								
			+				lymphosarcoma	ster, antib.
+								

Table 1

Nr.	Year	Author	Country	Age, sex	Race occupat. origin	A	Mycoses
90	1965	Gemeinhardt [35]	Germany	51, ♂			Candid. lung (C. alb.) Trichosp. cap. lung
91	1965	Gemeinhardt [35]	Germany	73, ♀			Candid. lung (C. alb.) Trichosp. cap. lung
92	1965	Perry et al. [67]	U.S.A.	58, ♂	white Texas cook		Histopl. lung Coccid. lung
93	1966	Brass, K. [15]	Venezuela	33, ♂		+	Phycom. lung, brain (M. corymbifer) Asp. lung + Cand. lung, + Kidney
94	1966	Rifkind et al. [74]	USA	17, ♂		+	Histopl. lung Aspergill. lung, brain P. carinii
95	1966	Rifkind et al. [74]	USA	40, ♂		+	Aspergill. lung P. carinii
96	1966	Rifkind et al. [74]	USA	38, ♂		+	Nocard. lung P. carinii
97	1966	Rifkind et al. [74]	USA	27, ♂		+	Aspergill. lung P. carinii
98	1966	Rifkind et al. [74]	USA	17, ♂		+	Nocard. lung P. carinii
99	1966	Symmers [100] (Symmers, 1965) [98]	Great Brit.	44, ♂		+	Cryptoc. skin, CNS lung Candid. dissemin. Asperg. dissemin. Phycom. lung, brain P. carinii (+++)
100	1966	Symmers [100]	Great Brit.				Cryptoc. (*) Candid. dissem. (*)
101 to 102	1966	Symmers [100]	Great-Brit.				Aspergill. dissem. Candid. dissemin.
103	1966	Symmers [100] Symmers [99]	Great Brit.	56, ♂		+	Phycom. dissemin. Candid. dissemin.
104	1966	Symmers [100]	Great Brit.				Aspergill. dissem. Candid. dissemin. Phycom. dissemin.
105 to 116	1966	Symmers [100]	Great Brit.				Asperg. dissemin. Phycom. dissemin.

(Continued)

Diagns. methods							Associated disease(s)	Treatment
H	B	Cam	Cpm	Ed	Im	In		
		+		+	+		Diabetes	Mycostatin, oral
		+		+	+			
		+		+	+			
		+		+	+			
		+			+		duodenal ulcer	Amphot. B (1.6 g)
		+			+			
+			+				Diabetes	
+								
+								
+							renal transplant	ster, antib, cytost.,
+								azathioprin
+								
+							renal transplant	thymectomy,
∅					+		sporozoan disease	splenectomy, irrad,
							cytomeg. vir. incl.	antib, ster, sulfam,
							of stomach	y globulins.
								azathioprin
+							renal transplant	ster, antib,
+							cytomeg. vir. lung	azathioprin
+							renal transplant	thymectomy,
+							Pseudom. lung	ster, antib,
								azathioprin
+							renal transplant	thymectomy
+							cytomeg. vir. lung	ster, antib,
								azathioprin
	+				+		Hodgkin, Tub, aden-	ster, cytost,
+							itis, cytomeg. vir.	irrad, antib,
+							lung, staphylo	lymphadenectomy
+							pyemia, blast cell	Nystat. local
+							leukemia	Amph. B
+			+				lymphat. leukemia	antib, ster,
+			+				staphylo abscess	cytost.
							of lung	

Table 1

Nr.	Year	Author	Country	Age, sex	Race occupat. origin	A	Mycoses
117	1967	Miyake and Okudaire [60]	Japan	14, ♂	japanese Kyushu	+	Cryptoc. dissemin. Candid. dissem.
118	1967	Miyake and Okudaire [60]	Japan	49, ♂	japanese Chugoku	+	Aspergill. lung Candid. dissemin.
119	1967	Miyake and Okudaire [60]	Japan	33, ♂	japanese Chugoku	+	Aspergill. lung Candid. esoph.
120	1967	Miyake and Okudaire [60]	Japan	82, ♀	japanese Kinki	+	Aspergill. lung Candid. esoph.
121	1967	Miyake and Okudaire [60]	Japan	48, ♂	japanese	+	Nocard. lung, esoph. Candid. lung
122	1967	Miyake and Okudaira [60]	Japan	42, ♀	japanese Kinki	+	Cryptoc. dissem. Geotrich, dissem.
123	1967	Miyake and Okudaira [60]	Japan	56, ♂	japanese Chubu	+	Aspergill. lung Phycom. lung
124	1967	Miyake and Okudaira [60]	Japan	40, ♂	japanese Kanto	+	Asperg. lung (A. fum.) Candid. lung (C. alb.)
125	1967	Miyake and Okudaira [60]	Japan	3, ♀	japanese Kanto	+	Aspergill. lung Candid. dig. tract
126	1967	Miyake and Okudaira [60]	Japan	64, ♂	japanese Kanto	+	Asperg. lung, trach. Candid. larynx
127	1967	Miyake and Okudaira [60]	Japan	53, ♀	japanese Kanto	+	Aspergill. intest. Candid. esoph., stomach
128	1967	Miyake and Okudaira [60]	Japan	60, ♂	japanese Kanto	+	Aspergill. lung Candid. esoph. col.
129	1967	Miyake and Okudaira [60]	Japan	71, ♀	japanese Kanto	+	Aspergill. lung Candid. dig. tract
130	1967	Miyake and Okudaira [60]	Japan	29, ♀	japanese Kanto	+	Cryptococc. dissem. Candid. esoph. duod.
131	1967	Miyake and Okudaira [60]	Japan			+	Cryptococc. (*) Candid. (*)
132	1967	Miyake and Okudaira [60]	Japan	20, ♂	japanese Kanto	+	Candid. esophag. Phycom. lung
133	1967	Miyaka and Okudaira [60]	Japan	59, ♂	japanese Kanto	+	Candid. stom. duod. Phycom. stom. duod.
134	1967	Miyaka and Okudaira [60]	Japan	22, ♀	japanese Kanto	+	Asperg. larynx, spleen Candid. app. vermif. Phycom. app. vermif.
135	1967	Miyake and Okudaira [60]	Japan	29, ♂	japanese Kanto	+	Cryptococc. dissem. Candid. Intest.
136	1967	Miyake and Okudaira [60]	Japan	20, ♀	japanese Tohoku	+	Asperg. lung, esoph. Candid. intest.

(Continued)

H	B	Cam	Cpm	Ed	Im	In	Associated disease(s)	Treatment
+								ster, antib,
+								
+							myeloid leukemia	antib
+								
+							chron. lymphat. leukemia	ster, antib.
+								
+							hypoplastic anemia	ster
+								
+							cancer of esophag	
+								
			+				monocytic leuk.	antib.
			+					
+							panmyelophtisis	antib, ster.
+								
			+				serum hepatitis severe emaciation (H-bomb test victim)	antib.
			+					
+					FAT		lymphat. leukemia	
+					FAT			
+							cancer of stomach, post-op. panperit. severe emaciation.	antib, ster.
+								
+							acute myeloid leuk. severe emaciation	antib, ster.
+								
+							myeloid leukemia	antib, ster.
			+					
+							myeloid leukemia	antib, ster.
+								
+							SLE	antib, ster.
+								
+					FAT		acute myeloid	
+					FAT		leukemia	
+							intestinal sarcoma, post-op. pan-peritonitis	
+								
+							severe emaciation	antib, ster.
+								
+								
+							monocyt. leukemia	antib, ster.
+								
+							myelosclerosis	antib, ster.
+								

Table 1

Nr.	Year	Author	Country	Age, sex	Race occupat. origin	A	Mycoses
137	1967	Miyake and Okudaira [60]	Japan	64, ♂	japanese Kanto	+	Aspergill. lung Candid. intest.
138	1967	Okudaira (x)	Japan	33, ♂	japanese Kanto	+	Aspergill. lung Candid. intest.
139	1967	Okudaira (x)	Japan	65, ♀	japanese Kanto	+	Aspergill. dissem. Phycom. lung, stom.
140	1967	Okudaira (x)	Japan	62, ♂	japanese Kanto	+	Aspergill. lung Phycom. dissem.
141	1967	Okudaira (x)	Japan	37, ♂	japanese Kanto	+	Aspergill. lung Candid. lung, esoph.
142	1967	Okudaira (x)	Japan	55, ♂	japanese Kanto	+	Aspergill. lung Phycom. dissemin.
143	1967	Okudaira (x)	Japan	3, ♂	japanese Kanto	+	Candid. esoph, stom. Phycom. esoph, stom.
144	1967	Peña [66]	Colombia	20, ♂	farmer	+	Histopl. dissem. Candid. esoph.
145	1967	Peña [66]	Colombia	15, ♂ d		+	Phycom. small bowel Candid. esoph.
146	1967	Pollak and Angulo o. [70]	Vene- zuela				Histopl. (*) Asperg. lung (A. fum.)
147		Salfelder and Schwarz (x)	U.S.A.			+	Cryptococc. CNS Pneum. car. (+)
148	1967 (1961)	Winn et al. [116] (Will et al.) [115]	U.S.A.	28, ♂	caucasian Californ.	+	Coccid. dissem. Asperg. dissem.
149	1968	Doehnert et al. [23]	Vene- zuela	9, ♀ m		+	Candid. lung P. carinii (++)
150	1968	Doehnert et al. [23]	Vene- zuela	17, ♀ m		+	Histopl. dissemin. P. carinii
151	1968	Doehnert et al. [23]	Vene- zuela	6, ♂ m		+	Histopl. primo-infec- tion P. carinii (+)
152	1968	Doehnert et al. [23]	Vene- zuela	3, ♀ m		+	Candid. lung P. carinii (++)
153	1968	Doehnert et al. [23]	Vene- zuela	7, ♀ m		+	Candid. lung. P. carinii (+)
154	1968	Drutz et al. [25]	U.S.A.	65, ♂	white	+	Histopl. dissemin. Nocard. lung (N. ast.)
155	1968	von Ledebur [50]	Switzer- land	40, ♂		+	Aspergill. lung Candid. digest. tr. CNS

(Continued)

H	B	Cam	Cpm	Ed	Im	In	Associated disease(s)	Treatment
+					FAT		cancer of stomach	
+					FAT			
+					FAT		acute myeloid leu-	
+					FAT		kemia	
+					FAT		agranulocytosis	
+					FAT			
+					FAT		cancer of stomach	
+					FAT			
+					FAT		generalised tub.	antib, ster.
+					FAT			
+					FAT		myeloid	antib, ster.
+					FAT		leukemia	
+					FAT		lymphatic leukemia	
+					FAT			
+	+							
+								
+							premature of 1.250 g	
							Tuberculosis	
+								
+								
+		+			+		lymphosarcoma	ster, antib, irrad
+		+					(Candid. oral)	cytost.
+							denutrition, anemia raquitism, broncho- pneumonia	
+								
+							anemia, intestinal parasites, denutrition, bronchopneum.	
+								
+							acute enterocolitis	
+								
+								
+								
+								
+								
∅		+					Diabetes, lympho-	Amphot. B, 2.301 g
+	+	+					sarcoma, congestive heart failure	Sulfonamide
+							delirium tremens	antib, ster.
+		+					hepatitis	
+								

Table 1

Nr.	Year	Author	Country	Age, sex	Race occupat. origin	A	Mycoses
156	1968	Leggat and de Kretser [51]	U.S.A.	47, ♂		+	Aspergill. lung (A. fum.) Candid. lung
157	1968	Pillay et al. [68]	U.S.A.	17, ♀	white	+	Histopl. lymph node Cryptoc. lung Candid. lung, skin
158	1968	Rocha Posada et al. [75]	Colombia	20, ♂	colored	+	Histopl. dissemin. Candid. esoph.
159	1968	Tynes et al. [104]	U.S.A.	64, ♂	white		Cryptoc. lung (?) Blastom. lung
160	1968	Tynes et al.	U.S.A.	51, ♂	white		Cryptoc. lung (?) Actinom. lung (?)
161	1969	Falcone and Garagusi [29]	U.S.A.	40, ♂	colored	+	Nocard. brain Sporotrich. dissem. cutan.
162	1969	Gerszten et al. [36]	U.S.A.	40, ♂	colored		Candid. lung Nocard. lung
163	1969	Gerszten et al. [36]	U.S.A.	10, ♀	colored	+	Candid. gastro-int Phycom. gastro-int
164	1969	McCarthy et al. [57]	Great Brit.	60, ♂	London-transport		Fungus-ball lung (Allesch. boydii) (Asperg. nidul.)
165	1969	Pedraza [65]	(Ohio, U.S.A.)			+	Histopl. dissem. Candid. stomach, liver
166	1969	Pedraza [65]	(Ohio, U.S.A.)			+	Phycom. (*) Asperg. (*)
167	1969	Pedraza [65]	(Ohio, U.S.A.)	4, ♂		+	Candid. (*) Geotrich. (*)
168	1969	Pedraza [65]	Colombia	4, m		+	Phycom. dissem. Asperg. lung
169	1969	Preisler et al. [71]	U.S.A.	36, ♂		+	Phycom. lung Candid. heart, tongue
170	1969	Preisler et al. [71]	U.S.A.	9, ♂		+	Aspergill. dissem. Candid. digest. tr. kidney (C. trop.)
171	1969	Preisler et al. [71]	U.S.A.	27, ♀		+	Aspergill. lung Candid. dissemin. (C. parapsil.)
172	1969	Preisler et al. [17]	U.S.A.	18, ♂		+	Aspergill. lung Candid. dissem.
173	1969	Preisler et al. [71]	U.S.A.	42, ♀		+	Aspergill. lung Candid. heart
174	1969	Preisler et al. [17]	U.S.A.	46, ♀		+	Aspergill. lung kidn. Candid. lung, kidn.

(Continued)

Diagns. methods							Associated disease(s)	Treatment
H	B	Cam	Cpm	Ed	Im	In		
+			+		+		spondylitis, tub?	irrad, antib, antitubercul.
+			+					
		+				+	SLE	ster, BUN
+			+					
		+	+					
+	+	+						
+								
		+						
		+						
		+						
		+					empyema	antib.
+	+	+	+				Boeck's sarcoid	ster, antib, KI
+	+	+						Amph. B, discontinued.
		+					rheumat. arthritis	
		+						
+							renal transplant	
+								
								antib.
	+	+			+			
	+	+			+			
	+							
	+							
+							leukemia	
+								
+			+				acute lymphat. leukemia	
+								
+								
+								
+							acute lymphoc. leukemia, Hodgkin	
+					+			
+							acute lymphocyt leukemia	Amph. B, 4 d. before death
+		+	+		+			
+							acute myelobl. leukemia, Klebsiella-septicemia	
+			+					
+							acute lymphocyt. leukemia, Klebsiella pneumonia	
+					+			
+							acute myeloid leukemia, Serratia	Amph. B, 8 d. before
			+		+			
+							acute lymphoc. leuk. Pseudom. in blood	
+								

Table 1

Nr.	Year	Author	Country	Age, sex	Race occupat. origin	A	Mycoses
175	1969	Preisler *et al.* [71]	U.S.A.	40, ♂		+	Aspergill. lung Candid. dissemin.
176	1969	Preisler *et al.* [71]	U.S.A.	43, ♂		+	Aspergill. lung Candid. lung, heart
177	1969	Preisler *et al.* [71]	U.S.A.	10, ♀		+	Aspergill. dissem. Candid. dissem.
178	1969	Preisler *et al.* [71]	U.S.A.	11, ♂		+	Aspergill. upper dig. tract, trachea Candid. stomach
179	1969	Rosen *et al.* [77]	U.S.A.	56. ♂		+	Monosporium lung (Allesch. boydii) Asperg. lung (A. fum.)
180	1969	Salfelder *et al.* [80]	Venezuela	46, ♂		+	Histopl. dissem. Paracocc. dissem.
181	1969	Salfelder *et al.* [80]	Venezuela	48, ♂		+	Histopl. lung, residual Paracocc. dissem.
182	1969	Salfelder (x) (E.35.980)	Venezuela	39, ♂			Paracocc. dissem. Chromo foot
183	1970	Brass [16]	Venezuela	15, ♀		+	Phycom. brain Histopl. lung, residual
184	1970	Salfelder (x) (A.4634)	Venezuela	30, ♂		+	Cryptoc. CNS Histopl. lung, residual Candid. lung
185	1970	Salfelder *et al.* [81]	Venezuela	2, ♂ m		+	Histopl. dissem. Candid. esoph.
186	1970	Salfelder *et al.* [81]	Venezuela	5, ♂		+	Histopl. dissem. Candid. lung.
187	1970	Schwarz (x) (A.6751)	U.S.A.	67, ♀	white	+	Histopl. lung, healed primary complex, Phycom. lung
188	1970	Schwarz (x) (A.6764)	U.S.A.	70, ♂	white	+	Histopl. lung, healed calcif. spleen Nocard. brain
189	1970	Schwarz (x) (A.6.800)	U.S.A.	73, ♂	negro	+	Phycom. lung Candid. stomach
190	1970	Schwarz (x) (A.6850)	U.S.A.	77, ♂	white	+	Nocard. lung, brain Candid. bladder Phycom. lung, brain

(Continued)

H	B	Cam	Cpm	Ed	Im	In	Associated disease(s)	Treatment
+							acute lymphoc. leuk.	
+					+			
+							acute lymphoc. leukemia	
+								
+			+				acute lymphocyt. leukemia	
+			+		+			
+							acute, myeloid leukemia, Escher. coli septicemia	
+								
+		+	+				ankylosing spondilitis	antib, intracavitary inj. of NaI.
		+						
+			+					
+							Chagas	
+								
+							dysenteric colitis	
+								
	+	+				+		amputation 3 fingers foot, for Chromo
	+							
+							Diabetes, glomerulo-nephritis	
+								
+							bacterial prostatitis, cachexia, intest. parasites	
+								
+								
+								
+								
+								
+								
+							multiple myeloma myeloma, carcinoma lung, anemia acute pyelonephr.	Talwin
+							bronchopneumonia hemorrh. cystitis, strepto meningit.	antib, ster, exploratory craniotomy
+								
+							gastrectomy, splen-ectomy, partial pan-createctomy for cancer, fecal peritonitis.	
+								
+							chron. lymphat. leu-kemia, carcinoma colon removed (7 y bef.), prostatect. (15 y bef.) Toxoplasmosis lung and brain, micronodul. ence-phalit., herpetic esopha-gitis cytomeg. vir. lung	cytost. (6 m) antib.
+								
+								

Table 1

Nr.	Year	Author	Country	Age, sex	Race occupat. origin	A	Mycoses
191	1970	Schwarz and Baum [85]	U.S.A.	48, ♂		+	Cryptococc. dissem. P. carinii
192	1970	Soper et al. [91]	U.S.A.	16, ♂			Coccidioid. lung Histopl. dissem.
193	1970	Young et al. [119]	U.S.A.				Asperg. dissem. Phycom. dissem.
194 to 197	1970	Young et al. [119]	U.S.A.			+	Asperg. dissem. Candid. dissem.

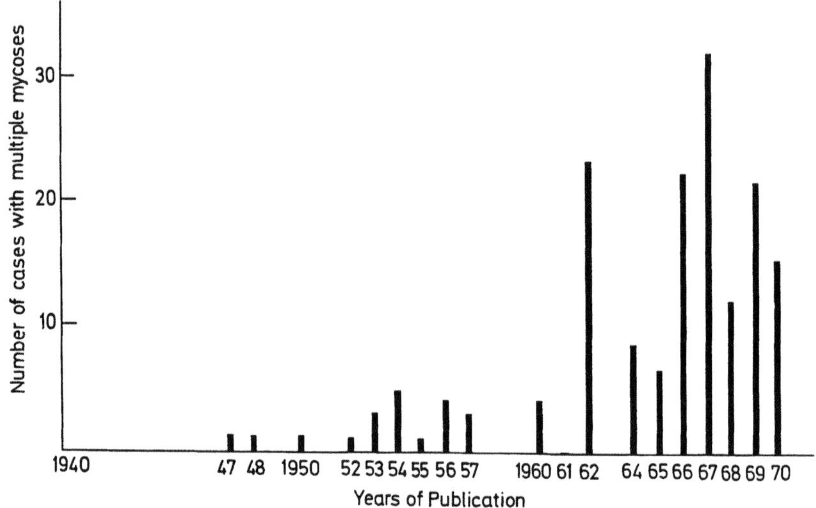

Table 2. Multiple Mycoses per Year

determination of the presence of septa is difficult if the hypha shows kinks and bends in tissue. This is true also if most hyphae seem to be without septa but one appears to be septate.

The identification of organisms of the genera *Candida* and *Aspergillus* in culture is simple but the interpretation is difficult. If one accepts any positive sputum culture containing one of the two above-mentioned genera as proof of pulmonary aspergillosis or candidosis, the incidence of these diseases will increase astronomically.

Age and sex were indicated in only 149 cases. Almost 50 percent of all patients were more than 45 years old (Table 3). Sex ratio was 96 male: 42 female.

Race: Data were given on race in 85 reports. On these, 47 were Caucasians, 28 Japanese, and 10 were described as "Negro" or "colored".

Table 3. Age groups

Years	Nr.
1– 9	6
10–19	16
20–29	17
30–39	15
40–49	19
50–59	28
60–69	23
70–79	25
80–89	6
90 +	3

(Continued)

Diagns. methods							Associated disease(s)	Treatment
H	B	Cam	Cpm	Ed	Im	In		
+	+	+		+				Amphot. B. Interrupted
+								
+					+			Amphot. B
+		+			+			
+		(+)						
+		(+)						

Table 4. Multiple mycoses-autopsies

Mycoses	Assoc. with 1 other M.	Assoc. with 2 or more other M	Autopsy			
			performed	supposedly performed	total	without autopsy
Candidosis	97	12	92	11	102 95%	5
Aspergillosis	89	7	74	5	78 84%	16
Phycomycosis	38	7	27	17	43 100%	
Histoplasmosis	39	5	31		31 72%	11
Cryptococcosis	30	7	28	4	32 87%	5
Pneumocystosis	19	5	24		24 100%	
Nocardiosis	12	2	12		12 86%	2
Blastomycosis	8		1		1 14%	7
Coccidioidomycosis	9		6		8 86%	2
Geotrichosis	6	1	2	5	7 100%	
Paracoccidioidomycosis	6	1	3		3 60%	3
Chromomycosis	2	1				3
Sporotrichosis	2	1	1		1	1
Mycetoma	1					1
Penicilliosis	1	1	2		2	
Trichosporosis	2					2
Monosporiosis	2		1		1	

Nota: Cases of actinomycosis not included.

10*

Occupation was rarely specified. Of the nine cases of reported occupations, five were farmers and the other four of different professions.

Multiple Associations and Concomitant Infections: These are listed in Tables 1, 4, 5, and 6 Mycoses found in association with each other were also those involved in multiple combinations. African histoplasmosis, Lobo's disease, rhinosporiodiosis were never reported as being found with other deep mycoses. Sixteen cases were reported in which three or more fungus infections occurred in the same patient. These are considered in a separate chapter, but are also commented on in the chapters on each entity.

Autopsies: In 136 cases — more than two thirds of all cases — autopsies were reported; in 32 others, the data in the reports permit the supposition that autopsies were performed. Necropsy was apparently performed in all cases of phycomycosis, pneumocystosis, sporotrichosis, monosporidiosis, and penicilliosis (Table 4).

C. Specific Entities

1. Candidosis

This was by far the most common coadunate organism, being found in association with one other mycosis in 97 cases and with two or more other mycoses in 11 instances. In 92 cases, necropsies were reported and are presumed to have been performed in 11 others.

Candidosis was disseminated in 31 cases (2, 3, 8, 14, 15, 37, 45, 57, 69, 70, 82, 99, 101–104, 117, 118, 155, 165, 170–172, 174–177, 194–197). In four cases, two organs were involved: in one, lung and skin (157) in two, lung and esophagus (23, 141), and in one, lung and kidney (93).

In the 56 cases involving a single organ, these included 18 in the lungs (5, 7, 46, 47, 83–87, 90, 91, 124, 149, 152, 153, 162, 184), 33 in the digestive tract (20–22, 24–26, 29, 41, 67, 68, 72, 119, 120, 125, 127–130, 132–138, 143–145, 158, 163, 178, 185, 189), one in the larynx (126), one in the bladder (190), two in the heart (169, 173), and one in the nose (73). Localization of the candidosis was not mentioned in 16 cases (50–61, 64, 100, 131, 167).

Associated mycoses were: aspergillosis in 54, cryptococcosis in 18, phycomycosis in 19, pneumocystosis in 9, histoplasmosis in 8, nocardiosis in 5, geotrichosis in 5, trichosporosis in 2, and penicilliosis in 1 case. No association of candidosis with blastomycosis, paracoccidioidomycosis, or coccidioidmycosis was reported.

No information on debilitating factors was available in 10 cases (100, 101, 104, 131, 165, 194–197). Eleven patients had no predisposing disease, but most had received some treatment (2, 3, 7, 45, 91, 117, 134, 152, 153, 158, 184). Patients with debilitating conditions included neoplasms in 63, renal affections in 5, of which 3 were transplants, bacterial infections in 9, diabetes in 4, of which steroid-induced hyperglycemia accounted for one, SLE in 1, tuberculosis in 1, anemia in 4, myelosclerosis in 2, hepatitis in 2, cytomegaly in 3, Fanconi's syndrome in 1, toxoplasmosis in 1, rickets in 1, and prematurity in 1 case.

Therapy in 51 patients included antibiotics (41), steroids (36), irradiation (9), cytostatics (14), azathioprin (2), kayquinone (1), iodides (1), lymphadenectomy (1), actinomycin C (1), amphotericin B (2) and other antifungal drugs (3).

The majority of cases were reported from the USA; other countries were Japan, Great Britain, Switzerland, Colombia, and Venezuela.

Ages ranged from 15 days to 82 years, the maximum number of cases occurring in the first, fourth, and sixth decades. Sex ratio was 51 males: 33 females.

Diagnosis of candidosis was made generally at autopsy by histology (2 with FAT). Cultures were made only exceptionally in autopsies. *Candida sp.* was rarely isolated during life, sometimes leading to diagnosis, sometimes not considered as causing the disease. In cultures, *C. albicans* was most often detected, although other species have also been found.

2. Aspergillosis

This mycosis was found associated with others in 95 cases, 7 of which showed more than two fungal infections. Autopsy was performed in 73 and is presumed to have been done in 5 others.

Aspergillosis was disseminated in 32 cases (8, 14, 76, 80, 82, 99, 101, 102, 104, 105–116, 134, 139, 148, 170, 174, 177, 193–197).

In 50 cases, it was localized in the lungs (5, 19, 21–23, 29, 30, 33–38, 41, 44, 66, 68, 69, 71, 72, 88, 89, 94, 95, 97, 118–120, 123–125, 128, 129, 137, 138, 140–142, 146, 153, 156, 164, 168, 171–173, 175, 176, 179); in one case each, in lung and trachea (126), in lung and esophagus (136), in trachea and digestive tract (178), in the brain (42), in the intestine (127), and in the myocardium (43). Localization was not mentioned in 7 cases (50–55, 166).

In the cases with pulmonary involvement, diffuse lesions were observed in 16 (19, 21–23, 29, 37, 76, 95, 146, 155, 171–176). Twelve infections were tumorous, 11 of these forming fungus balls (5, 30, 33–36, 41, 44, 66, 156, 164, 179). Debilitating conditions were present in all diffused cases but not in the tumorous lesions.

Associated mycoses were: candidosis, 26; phycomycosis, 26; histoplasmosis, 8; pneumocystosis, 7; nocardiosis, 2; monosporiosis, 2; and penicilliosis, coccidioidomycosis, and cryptococcosis in 1 case each. No associations were found with blastomycosis, paracoccidioidomycosis, mycetoma, geotrichosis, and trichosporosis. No data on associated diseases was provided in 21 cases (101, 102, 104, 105–116, 168, 193–197).

Debilitating diseases were not found associated with aspergillosis in 5 cases; other patients had the following predisposing disorders: neoplasm in 45, renal transplants in 4, bacterial infection in 7, diabetes in 1, tuberculosis in 2, sporozoan disease in 1, hepatitis in 3, myelosclerosis in 2, anemia in 3, agranulocytosis in 2, spondylitis in 2, panmyelophtisis in 1, ulcerative colitis in 1, Cushing'disease in 1, and cytomegaly in 1 case.

Therapy was reported for 43 patients: antibiotics in 40, steroids in 32, cytostatics in 7, azathioprin in 4, thymectomy in 2, splenectomy in 1, adrenalectomy in 1, lymphadenectomy in 1, irradiation in 8, iodides in 2, actinomycin C in 1, ACTH in 1, amphotericin B in 3, and other antifungal drugs in 2.

Ages ranged from 4 months to 82 years, most patients being in their forties and sixties. The male: female ratio was 2:1. The majority of cases were from the USA; others were reported from Japan, Great Britain, Switzerland, Venezuela and Colombia.

Pulmonary fungus balls were found in most cases diagnosed during life, the diagnosis being made by x-ray or after surgery. Almost all other cases of aspergillosis were diagnosed at autopsy. Some patients had positive cultures, usually of *A. fumigatus*, during life, but these were not considered diagnostic unless the fungus was repeatedly isolated. In two additional cases, not listed in Table 1, two or three species of Aspergillus were isolated from different lesions of the same patient: *A. fumigatus* in the lung and *A. glaucus* in the spleen in one (Young *et al.* [119]), and *A. flavus* in the myocardium and *A. fumigatus* and *A. nidulans* in the lung in another (Welsch and Buchness [113]).

3. Phycomycosis

Phycomycosis was found in association with one or more mycoses in 44 cases; in 27 of these there is evidence of necropsies and it is assumed that autopsies were performed in the remainder.

Twenty-one cases were disseminated (25, 26, 41, 103–116, 140, 142, 168, 172): 6 in lungs (42, 123, 132, 169, 187, 189); 1 in lung and spleen (24); 4 in lung and brain (71, 93, 99, 190); 3 in brain (65, 73, 183); 1 in lung and stomach (139); 5 in the digestive tract (133, 134, 143, 145, 162) and 3 with sites of involvement not reported (61, 69, 166). Associated mycoses included: aspergillosis, 27 (41, 42, 71, 93, 99, 104, 116, 123, 134, 139, 140, 142, 166, 168, 190, 193), candidosis, 18 (24–26, 41, 61, 73, 99, 103, 104, 132–134, 143, 145, 162, 169, 190), cryptococcosis, 3 (62, 65, 99), histoplasmosis, 2 (69, 183), nocardiosis, 1 (190), geotrichosis, 1 (69) and pneumocystosis, 1 (99).

In 15 cases no information is available about associated diseases. In the other 28 patients, only one was not reported to have a debilitating disease (134). Pathologic conditions were: 20 neoplastic disease (71%); 3 were renal affections; 4, diabetes; 3, hematologic disorders; 2 cytomegaly; and 1 each toxoplasmosis, tuberculosis, and prematurity.

Treatment, mentioned in only 9 cases, consisted of antibiotics, steroids, cytotoxics, and radiotherapy.

Ages ranged from one premature neonate of 15 days to 77 years. The highest number of infections occurred during the 5th decade. Sex is mentioned in 26 instances: 16 males and 10 females. Phycomycosis is worldwide in distribution. In this series, 16 cases were reported from Europe, 8, 15 by Symmers in Great Britain, but most without details; 16 from U.S.A.; from Japan; and 4 from South America (2 Colombia and 2 Venezuela).

Diagnosis was made in all cases but one (73) at necropsy. Lack of diagnosis made during life was due, first, to the fact that attention was focused on the primary disease; however, a sudden change of symptoms should suggest secondary fungal infection. Second, evolution of fungus infection was rapid (from a few days to a month.). Finally, positive cultures were difficult to obtain. Only in 4 cases (25, 41, 42, 93) *Mucor sp.* grew in postmortem cultures, while in the only case diagnosed during life, *Rhizopus sp.* had grown.

Culture work being so problematic, diagnosis had to rely quite exclusively on morphology in histologic sections of broad hyphae, irregular in width and without septa.

4. Histoplasmosis

Forty-four cases of histoplasmosis were found associated with other mycoses. Autopsy had been performed in 31 of them. The disseminated form of the disease was present in 14 cases (1, 4, 6, 28, 45, 144, 150, 154, 158, 165, 180, 186, 192). Sixteen patients had active lung infection (9, 27, 33–36, 38, 40, 77–81, 92, 94), while in one, only the adrenals (11) and in another, only lymph nodes were found with histoplasmic lesions (157).

Ten cases showed residual lung lesions (16–18, 30, 75, 181, 183, 184, 187, 188) and in two (12, 146) no information of localization was available.

Other mycoses in association with histoplasmosis were: cryptococcosis, 10 (1, 4, 9, 11, 12, 27, 28, 45, 157, 184); candidosis, 8 (44, 144, 157, 158, 165, 184–186); blastomycosis, 7 (6, 40, 77–81); aspergillosis, 8 (30, 33–36, 38, 94, 146); coccidioidomycosis, 6 (75, 92, 192); pneumocystosis, 3 (27, 94, 150); paracoccidioidomycosis, 2 (154, 188); nocardiosis, 2 (154, 188); phycomycosis, 2 (183, 187).

Five cases presented triple mycotic infection (27, 45, 94, 157, 184).

Associated diseases were not reported in 15 patients. The others suffered from the following disorders: neoplasm 6; bacterial infection, 7; tuberculosis, 3; renal affections, 5 (one transplant); intestinal parasitosis, 3; diabetes, 2; SLE, 1; anemia, 4; peptic ulcer, 2; and Chagas' disease, 1; arthritis, cerebral hemorrhage, and cardiopathy, 1 each.

Treatment was reported in only a few cases: antibiotics in 4, steroids in 6, cytotoxics in 1, stilbamidine in 2, and irradiation in 2. Four patients treated with amphotericin B.

Ages varied from 2 months to 81 years, with a maximum in the 4th decade. All patients but four were males.

Histoplasmosis is one of the ubiquitous mycoses, with infections occurring in a high percentage of the population living in endemic areas. So it is not surprising that 33 cases of this series were reported from the USA nearly all from endemic regions, 7 from Venezuela, and 2 from Colombia. In the 27 autopsy cases from Japan, none had histoplasmosis or residual lesions of this fungal disease.

In disseminated histoplasmosis, a diagnosis was made before death in only

5 cases (4 from USA and 1 from Colombia), either by biopsy, direct examination, or sputum culture.

In the remaining cases (4 from Venezuela), diagnosis was made at autopsy.

In the 18 cases with localized histoplasmic, mostly pulmonary, lesions, 12 were diagnosed during life, using the above mentioned techniques and in addition immunologic methods.

Diagnosis of the residual lung lesions was based on autopsy findings.

It is to be emphasized that residual calcified mycotic foci occur only in histoplasmosis and coccidioidomycosis, never in other deep mycoses. They may, however, represent residual foci of tuberculosis. The finding of residual histoplasmotic lung foci at necropsy in highly endemic areas of histoplasmosis is so frequent (when looked for) that other fungal infections in these cases are only coincidental and not true multiple fungus infections. All known facts reinforce the belief that reactivation of inactive foci with secondary dissemination (endogenous reinfection) occurs only rarely.

5. Cryptococcosis

Thirty-seven cases of cryptococcosis were associated with other mycoses. Autopsy was done in 28 cases and may be supposed to have been done in 4 more.

Seventeen were disseminated (1, 2, 10, 12, 13, 15, 27, 45, 49, 64, 85, 99, 117, 122, 130, 135, 191), while 6 showed exclusive lung involvement (28, 31, 84, 157, 159, 160), 5, involvement of the CNS (3, 11, 39, 147, 184), 1 of lungs and CNS (32), and 1 each of skin (4), and of bones (7). In 6 patients, localization of cryptococcosis was not mentioned (9, 59–61, 100, 131).

Other mycoses associated with cryptococcosis were, in order of frequency: candidosis, 17 (2, 3, 7, 15, 59–61, 84, 85, 99, 100, 117, 130, 131, 135, 157, 184); histoplasmosis, 10 (1, 4, 9, 11, 12, 27, 28, 45, 157, 184); pneumocystosis, 6 (27, 31, 49, 99, 147, 191); phycomycosis, 3 (61, 64, 99); nocardiosis, 2 (13, 49); and blastomycosis (159), coccidioidomycosis (10), aspergillosis (99), geotrichosis (122), paracoccidioidomycosis (32), and mycetoma (39) 1 each. In one case (160), *A. israeli* had been cultured from sputum, but apparently there was no actinomycosis.

Six cases had more than two mycoses (27, 49, 63, 99, 157, 184).

Associated diseases were not reported in 3 cases and reported as not present in 9 others. The 25 included 12 with neoplasms, 4 with tuberculosis, 3 with bacterial infections, 3 with anemia, 2 each with SLE, renal affections, intestinal parasitosis, and cytomegaly, and 1 each with microangiopathy, hepatopathy, and toxoplasmosis. Some of these patients had several diseases.

Three cases presented the association of cryptococcosis, Hodgkin's disease, and tuberculosis with one or more other mycoses.

Antibiotics, in 12; steroids, in 8; cytotoxics, and irradiation, in 4 including 1 case each with stilbamidine and tuberculostatic drugs and 3 cases with amphotericin B.

Ages ranged from 4 to 66 years, most frequently in the 30 to 50 year age group.

In younger patients there is a peak between 10 and 20 years.

Sex ratio was 24:7 male: female, in the 31 cases in which sex was indicated.

Twenty-five cases, with associated mycoses were reported from the USA, 5 from Japan, 3 from Great Britain, and 2 each from Venezuela and Brazil. No cases with multiple fungus infections were reported from Australia or Continental Europe, despite the numerous case reports of cryptococcosis in these countries.

Fifteen cases were diagnosed during life by culture, direct examination (sputum, spinal fluid, and biopsy of skin lesions), but unhappily, in many of these cases, only in the terminal stage of life, when symptoms of meningitis were already present.

When cryptococcosis was recognized during life, in the majority of cases the other mycoses were also diagnosed.

In the cases with diagnosis at autopsy, positive cultures had been obtained in five. In six other cases, no details are known by what means, other than histologic, diagnosis was established.

6. Pneumocystosis

This parasite has a questionable place among fungi; nevertheless its behavior (and structure) simulates that of certain "opportunistic" fungi. Pneumocystosis was associated 24 times with mycoses (27, 32, 46, 48, 49, 66, 86–89, 94–99, 147, 149–153, 191). Autopsy was reported in all cases. The degree of involvement mentioned by authors ranges from the pauciparasitic form (+) to massive invasion (+ + + +).

All reports deal with pneumocystic lung infections, despite recent descriptions of extrapulmonary pneumocystic lesions (JARNUM *et al.* [44], BARNETT *et al.* [7]).

Mycoses found in association with these microorganism were: candidosis 9 (46–48, 86, 87, 99, 149, 152, 153); aspergillosis: 7 (66, 88, 89, 94, 95, 97, 99); cryptococcosis: 6 (27, 31, 49, 99, 147, 191); histoplasmosis: 4 (27, 94, 150, 151); nocardiosis: 3 (49, 96, 98); phycomycosis: 1 (99); and penicilliosis: 1 (86). In 5 cases there were two or more mycoses associated with pneumocystosis (27, 49, 86, 94, 99). Debilitating diseases were absent in 2 cases (152, 191) and were not known in a third (147). In the other 21 patients, associated diseases were; neoplasms in 9, renal transplants in 5, acute colitis and anemia with malnutrition and intestinal parasitism (in minors) in 2 each, and anemia and angiopathy, 1 each.

Treatment was given in all cases of cancer and consisted of antibiotics, steroids, cytotoxics, and/or irradiation. In cases of renal transplants, antibiotics, steroids, and azathioprin were administered. Children under 1 year of age did not receive treatment.

Two age groups were involved: 9 children under age 10 and adults, the majority over 40 years of age. Males numbered 14 and females 9,.

In all cases but one (92), diagnosis was made at autopsy. In this single case — pneumocystosis and aspergillosis after renal transplant — organisms of *P. carinii* had been found in tracheal aspirate. At autopsy, however, no parasites were found and it is assumed that pneumocystosis had healed.

Associated pulmonary mycoses have been found in pneumocystosis from cortisone injections in rats (SETHI *et al.* [87]).

7. Nocardiosis

Nocardiosis was found associated with other mycoses in 14 cases. In twelve, autopsy had been performed. Disseminated disease was found in only two (49, 83). Of the remaining cases, 8 were pulmonary infections (14, 43, 44, 67, 94, 96, 154, 162), 1 with lung and brain involvement (190); 2 with exclusive brain infection (161, 188); and 1 without detailed information (63).

Associated mycoses included candidosis; 5 (63, 67, 83, 162, 190); aspergillosis: 3 (43, 44, 190); pneumocystosis: 3 (49, 93, 95); cryptococcosis: 2 (13, 49); histoplasmosis: 2 (154, 188); phycomycosis: 1 (190) and sporotrichosis: 1 (161). No association with blastomycosis, coccidioidimycosis, paracoccidioidomycosis, chromomycosis, or geotrichosis was reported. Two cases presented more than 2 mycoses (49, 190).

Most patients had at least one associated disorder, including 8 with neoplasms, 2 with diabetes, and 1 each with toxoplasmosis, bacterial meningitis, and colitis. Three were associated with renal transplants. Antibiotics were given in all cases, and, in addition, steroids in 6 patients, cytotoxic agents in 2 and radiotherapy in one.

Ages ranged from 17 to 77 years, with a maximum in the 3rd decade. Males predominated in a ratio of 12:2. All cases were reported in the USA, although nocardia is ubiquitous.

Diagnosis was made during life in 3 cases (151, 158, 159), 3 by biopsy and 2 of them, in addition, by culture. The other mycoses in these cases were also found before death, while in all the other cases, mycoses were diagnosed at necropsy. Most necropsy cases were diagnosed histologically, only a few being corroborated by culturing. In all reported cultures, the causative agent was *N. asteroides*.

8. Blastomycosis

Of 8 cases of blastomycosis, autopsy was performed in only one. One case (6) was disseminated; 6 cases were confined to the lungs (40, 70, 77, 78, 81, 159); and fungal lesions were found in lungs and skin in 1 case (79).

Only 2 mycoses were associated with blastomycosis: in 6 cases, histoplasmosis and in 1 case, possible cryptococcosis (159). No cases with more than two mycoses were detected.

Debilitating diseases, present in 3 cases were: duodenal ulcer, arthritis, and pulmonary tuberculosis. The only patient in whom chemotherapy may have played a contributory role was a 39-year-old man with a 3-year history of steroid administration. Ages ranged from 43 to 74 years, with 50% during the 4th decade. All patients were male, 3 were farmers, 1 was a seaman, and 1 was a machinist; the occupations of the other three is not known.

In 7 patients diagnosis was made in vivo by culture, immunology, biopsy, or inoculation, the majority of positive diagnosis resulting from cultures of sputum. In all these cases the associated mycoses were diagnosed also in vivo.

All patients had lived in endemic areas in the USA. Formerly, North America was the only continent in which blastomycosis was known to occur. Recently, however autochthonous infections have been reported from Africa (CAMPOS DE MAGELHAES [18], EMMONS *et al.* [26]).

9. Coccidioidomycosis

Nine cases of coccidioidomycosis were reported in this series; six with autopsy. Five were active coccidioidal infections: one disseminated (148), three localized to the lungs (65, 92, 192), and one believed to be also a pulmonary infection (10). The four remaining cases showed residual lesions (16–18, 75).

The cases with active lesions were associated with cryptococcosis (10), histoplasmosis (92, 192), aspergillosis (148), and actinomycosis (65). The four patients with residual lung lesions all showed also residual pulmonary foci of histoplasmosis (16–18, 75).

Debilitating conditions were present in three of the active forms of coccidioidomycosis: hepatopathy with uremia, duodenal ulcer, and lymphosarcoma. Only in the case of lymphosarcoma (145) was treatment mentioned: antibiotics, steroids, radiation, and cytostatics.

In 1 case (65), no mention is made of predisposing factors. Patients ranged in age from 16 to 81 years, with the average in the 5th decade. All were men. Occupations were not mentioned. Racially, 2 patients were Caucasian and 1 was black.

Nearly all patients had lived in endemic areas of the USA: Arizona, California, Nevada, New Mexico, and Utah.

This geographical limitation leads to correct diagnosis in a patient with adequate symptoms, even if he is seen abroad (SYMMERS [96]).

Diagnosis was made during life by immunology and culture in three of the active mycoses (92, 148, 192). The residual lesions were found at necropsy in an epidemiologic research study (STRAUB and SCHWARZ [94], SCHWARZ *et al.* [86]).

10. Geotrichosis

Seven cases of geotrichosis are reported (55–58, 62, 122, 167). Necropsies were reported in only two, but it is assumed that all were autopsied. Two cases (122, 167) were disseminated infections, while in the others, localization of the lesions is not known.

Associated mycoses were: candidosis: 5 (55–58, 167), cryptococcosis: 1 (122); phycomycosis: 1 (64); and aspergillosis: 1 (55). In one case (55) a triple fungus infection was found.

Seven cases involved neoplastic disorders. Hutter and Collins [43] mention cancer in five of their patients (55–58, 62). In two other cases (122, 167) leukemia was cited. Six cases were from the USA and one from Japan.

In one case (119) diagnosis was made after necropsy by culture and probably the same occurred in another case (164). No information is available on whether diagnosis of the 5 remaining cases was made by histology. Age and sex were reported in only 2 cases, one, a woman aged 42 and one, a boy aged 4 years.

Geotrichosis is a somewhat rare disease of somewhat shaky standing; we have never identified this condition in any of our own material. It should be pointed out that, of the several thousand species of fungi, each and every one can conceivably become an "opportunistic invader", and the interpretation in every individual case should be made with caution. For example, species of *Candida* and *Torulopsis* are not infrequently isolated from the blood of patients with indwelling intravenous catheters; not only have we seen "fungus thrombi" in the lumina of the catheters, which produce infusion of yeasts into the bloodstream; we have also seen spontaneous disappearance of the fungemia after removal of the catheter.

11. Paracoccidioidomycosis

Six paracoccidioidal infections from the literature and from our material, have been found associated with other mycoses. In three of these autopsy was performed.

Four showed disseminated disease (32, 180–182), one involved the lungs and oral cavity (74), and one showed only lung lesions at the time of diagnosis (19).

Associated mycoses were: chromomycosis: 3 (19, 74, 182); histoplasmosis: 2 (180, 181); cryptococcosis: 1 (32); and sporotrichosis: 1 (19). One (19) had a triple mycotic infection.

Associated disorders, present in 4 cases, were those expected in less-developed countries: two with tuberculosis, intestinal parasitosis and anemia, one with dysenteric colitis, and one with Chagas' disease. None of these conditions was treated. Four cases were from Venezuela, one from Costa Rica, and one from Brazil. All were men and ages range from 39 to 54 years.

In 4 patients, the paracoccidioidal infection was diagnosed during life, by biopsy and culture, direct examination of sputum and inoculation of sputum into animals. In one of these patients (32), a second mycosis was overlooked at the time the paracoccidioidomycosis was detected.

12. Chromomycosis

Three cases of cutaneous chromomycosis, all associated with paracoccidioidomycosis, have been published (19, 74, 182). No autopsy was performed in any of these cases. Case 19 had also sporotrichosis. In all patients, the chromomycosis was diagnosed several years before paracoccidioidomycosis or sporotrichosis was found. The chromomycosis was untreated in two cases (19, 74) and led to amputation in the third (182).

One case (74) was associated with tuberculosis, anemia, and intestinal parasitosis.

All three patients were men, aged 39, 46, 54, respectively. The cases were reported from Brazil, Costa Rica, and Venezuela.

Diagnosis was made by biopsy and direct examination of pus. The typical morphology of the dark-brown fungus cells permits diagnosis of the disease, but only by culture (not made in these cases) can the causative species, of several that produce this disease, be determined.

13. Sporotrichosis

Two cases of sporotrichosis with cutaneous manifestations were found associated with other fungus infections, nocardiosis (161) in 1 case, chromomycosis and paracoccidioidomycosis in the other (19). In 1 case (161) autopsy was performed.

Associated disease was Boeck's sarcoidosis in 1 case (161). The patient, a man aged 40, had received antibiotics and steroids. In the other case no mention is made of associated disease or treatment.

One case (19) was reported from Brazil; the other (161) was from the USA. Sporotrichosis is known to be ubiquitous.

All mycoses were diagnosed in vivo by biopsy and culture.

Histologic diagnosis alone of sporotrichosis may be difficult, because of scarcity of fungus cells in the tissues, but fungi grow easily on culture media and can be seen in animal tissues after inoculation of suspicious material.

14. Mycetoma

One case of mycetoma of an ankle in association with cryptococcosis (39) was diagnosed by biopsy and culture (*Madurella grisea*). No debilitating disease was present and no drugs had been given, other than those to combat both fungi: stilbamidine, amphotericin B, and X5079C. The patient, a North American farmer aged 61, responded to treatment.

15. Actinomycosis

One case of double mycosis was found in the literature (165): cervical actinomycosis was associated with coccidioidomycosis of lungs. Another case (160) represented *A. israeli* in the sputum but actinomycosis was not found.

16. Rare Mycoses

In two cases *Penicillium sp.* was found: in one with aspergillosis (76) and in one, with candidosis and pneumocystosis (86). Both were found at autopsy.

Debilitating disease in the first patient was terminal bacterial septicemia and in the second, stem cell leukemia. Both were boys under age 10 and both were reported from the U.S.A. Diagnosis was made in one during life by biopsy and subsequent culture; in the other case, *Penicillium sp.* was cultured post-mortem.

Superficial penicilliosis is rare, and the role of *Penicillium sp.* as a pathogen in viscera, when found only in cultures, is questionable.

Gemeinhardt [35] reported two patients (90, 91) with pulmonary symptoms. Culture of sputum revealed both *Trichosporum capitatum* and *Candida sp.* In a close follow-up study, he concludes that both fungi were responsible for the disease. The patients were a man of 51 and a woman aged 73 years, of whom the man had diabetes. Both lived in Germany. Diagnosis was by culture, immunology tests, and direct examination of sputum.

In 2 other cases (164 and 179), fungus ball of the lung in one contained *Monosporium apiospermium* (Allescheria boydii) and *Aspergillus sp.*; in the other, *Aspergillus fumigatus* was found. Autopsy was performed in one (179).

In one case (164), a 60-year-old man living in Great Britain, there was no associated disease and the patient had received only antibiotics. Diagnosis was made in vivo by biopsy, culture, and immunology.

The second patient (179) was a man of 56 years with spondylitis; the only drugs administrated before his pulmonary disease were antibiotics. This case was reported from the U.S.A. Diagnosis was made during life by culture and confirmed at necropsy.

17. More Than Two Mycoses

(Table 5)

Sixteen cases were found with more than 2 mycoses; 15 had triple (19, 27, 41, 45, 49, 55, 61, 86, 93, 94, 104, 134, 157, 184, 190) and one (99) a quintuple mycotic infection. Autopsy was performed in all.

In 5 patients, 2 or more mycoses were disseminated (45, 49, 99, 104, 190); in 6 others, 1 mycosis was disseminated or localized in at least 2 different systems (27, 41, 93, 94, 134, 157).

Of the 16 patients, 12 had candidosis, 7 aspergillosis, 7 phycomycosis, 6 cryptococcosis, 5 pneumocystosis, 4 histoplasmosis (two of them residual lesions), 2 nocardiosis and 1 each geotrichosis, penicilliosis, paracoccidioidomycosis, chromomycosis and sporotrichosis.

The same association of fungus infections (candidosis-aspergillosis-phycomycosis) was found in 4 cases (41, 93, 104, 134) and, in a fifth (99), was found associated with cryptococcosis and pneumocystosis.

Table 5. Cases involving more than 2 mycoses

Case Nr.	Cand.	Asp.	Phyco.	Crypto.	P. car.	Histo.	Noc.	Parac.	Chromo.	Sporo.	Geot.	Peni.
19								lung	foot	finger		
27				dis.	+	res.						
41	esoph.	lung	dis.									
45	dis.			dis.		dis.						
49				dis.	+		dis.					
55*	+	+									+	
61*	+		+	+								
86	lung				+							+
93	lung kidn.	lung	lung brain									
94		lung brain			+	lung						
99	dis.	dis.	lung brain	dis. A = lung	+							
104*	dis.	dis.	dis.									
134	app. verm.	lar. spleen	app. verm.									
157	lung skin			lung			lymph node					
184	lung			brain		res.						
190	bladd.		lung brain					lung brain				
Total	12	7	7	6	5	4	2	1	1	1	1	1

* Case without detailed information.
dis. = disseminated; res. = residual; A. = Autopsy.

Debilitating factors were overwhelmingly frequent in this group, often
several existing in one patient. In 1 patient (134) no associated disease was
found at autopsy, but the patient had been treated for a suspected Wegener's
granulomatosis. Another case has no mention of associated diseases (93).
Only 2 cases (44, 101) are without information in this respect.

Of the 12 patients with one or more nonmycotic disorder, 6 had neoplasm,
1 was a renal transplant, and 1 each had diabetes, SLE, and bacterial prosta-
titis with intestinal parasitosis. Case 99 had Hodgkin's disease, tuberculosis,
leukemia, bacterial pneumonia, and cytomegaly; patient 190 had leukemia,
intestinal carcinoma, toxoplasmosis, herpetic esophagitis, and cytomegaly.

In the 8 cases for which treatment is mentioned, antibiotics were given in 7,
steroids in 6, cytotoxics in 7, irradiation in 1, tuberculostatic drugs in 1;
lymphadenectomy had been performed in 1 and amphotericin B given in 2.

In the 2 cases with multiple nonmycotic disorders (99, 190), high doses of several drugs had been administered, and the patient of case 99 had been given irradiation. Thus, it is imposible to incriminate one particular factor (disease and/or treatment) as predisposing to fungus disease.

Ages ranged from 9 to 77 years, with a 10:3 male predominance.

Ten cases were from the U.S.A., 2 from Great Britain, 1 from Japan, 2 from Venezuela, and 1 from Brazil.

Three mycoses were diagnosed during life in 1 case (19). Two mycoses were diagnosed in 2 cases (45, 157), and one mycosis in another (99). In all the remaining patients (the great majority), all mycoses were necropsy findings.

18. Associated Mycoses

Factors in the determination of association appear to be primarily such debilitating conditions as associated disease or chemotherapy, geographic regions, or diathesis. In 11 cases, two or more mycoses or fungal infections were found in association. Associations with less than two cases were not considered (Table 6).

The largest number of associations occurred in candidosis, aspergillosis, phycomycosis, and cryptococcosis with frequent combination between these mycoses themselves. The most frequent association was between candidosis and aspergillosis, followed by aspergillosis and phycomycosis, both fungus elements being active invaders of blood-vessel walls.

Disseminated forms were observed frequently in these four mycoses and their associations: in candidosis-aspergillosis, 21; aspergillosis-phycomycoses, 38; and in candidosis-cryptococcosis, 5.

In the association candidosis-aspergillosis, dissemination of both 8 times. In aspergillosis-phycomycosis dissemination of both was seen 16 times and dissemination of phycomycosis alone 6 times. In candidosis-cryptococcosis dissemination of both mycoses occurred in all cases.

Nocardiosis and geotrichosis showed relatively frequent association with candidosis. Almost no association was found between aspergillosis and crypto-coccosis, phycomycosis and cryptococcosis, or phycomycosis and pneumo-cystosis.

Association with pneumocystosis was limited to the six more frequent mycoses, mostly as pauciparasitic and paucireactive final infection with *P. carinii*.

These six mycoses should be put into one group, since they occurred with great frequency in patients with debilitating disorders; with histoplasmosis, blastomycosis, coccidioidomycosis, and paracoccidioidomycosis, this was not the case, or at least to a very minor degree. While these were found less often than any others except histoplasmosis their occurrence must be considered in the light of their geographic distribution, exacerbated by international travelling. The especially large number of cases associated with histoplasmosis is due in part to the frequency of residual and inactive lesions in areas where

Table 6. Associated mycoses

	Cand.	Asp.	Phyco.	Histo.	Crypto.	Pneum.	Nocard.	Blasto.	Cocci.	Geotr.	Parac.	Chromo
and.		48+(6)	11+(7)	5+(3)	13+(4)	7+(2)	4+(1)	—	(1)	4+(1)	—	—
.sp.	48+(6)		21+(6)	7+(1)	(1)	5+(2)	2+(1)	—	(1)	(1)	—	—
'hyco.	11+(7)	21+(6)		2	1+(2)	(1)	(1)	—	—	1	—	—
[isto.	5+(3)	7+(1)	2		7+(3)	2+(2)	2	7	6	—	2	—
rypto.	13+(4)	(1)	1+(2)	7+(3)		3+(3)	1+(1)	1	—	1	1	—
'neumo.	7+(2)	5+(2)	(1)	2+(2)	3+(3)		2+(1)	—	—	—	—	—
[ocard.	4+(1)	2+(1)	(1)	2	1+(1)	2+(1)		—	—	—	—	—
;lasto.	—	—	—	7	1	—	—		—	—	—	—
.occi.	(1)	(1)	—	6	1	—	—	—		—	—	—
;eotr.	4+(1)	(1)	1	—	1	—	—	—	—		—	—
'ara.	—	—	—	2	1	—	—	—	—	—		2+(1)
;hromo.	—	—	—	—	—	—	—	—	—	—	2+(1)	

): More than the two mycoses.

histoplasmosis is endemic, other mycoses often being acquired years after such primary infection with histoplasmosis. To a minor degree, this applies also to residual lesions in coccidioidomycosis. It should be kept in mind that residual lesions-with calcifications occur with any degree of regularity only in histoplasmosis and coccidioidomycosis, while in other mycoses such lesions are rare.

Local predisposition could be considered as a factor in combinations between histoplasmosis and aspergillosis, with formation of fungus balls in histoplasmotic cavitary lesions.

Sequence of infections can be determined in only 47 cases. The first occurring mycotic infection was detected in 35 cases. There is sufficient evidence to assume that infection with *H. capsulatum* was first in 17 cases; in 6 cases (30, 33–36, 38) fungus balls developed in previously existing cavities; in 1 case (146), aspergillosis was evidently a secondary infection. In 6 other cases (27, 181, 183, 184, 187, 188) the residual foci of histoplasmosis were definitely older lesions, on histologic grounds, than those of the other mycoses.

Further, in 4 cases of residual histoplasmic and coccidial lesions (16–18, 75), the patients were known to have lived first in histoplasmosis endemic areas.

In two additional cases (154, 157), the authors themselves assert that histoplasmosis had been acquired first.

In 5 cases (3, 31, 99, 147, 191), cryptococcosis apparently was the first infection, as it had been diagnosed first in vivo. In 5 cases of chromomycosis, mycetoma, and sporotrichosis (19, 39, 74, 161, 182), the chronicity of these mycotic infections suggests their earlier presence. In 7 cases — 6 of histoplasmosis and 1 of paracoccidioidomycosis (150, 151, 158, 165, 180, 185, 186) — the authors considered these mycoses to have been present first.

In 12 instances, we believed that fungal infections took place simultaneously: in 5 cases with *H. capsulatum* and *B. dermatitidis* (77–81), in two with *H. capsulatum* and *Cr. neoformans* (1, 4), in one with *H. capsulatum* and *C. immitis* (92), in two with aspergillus and *All. boydii* (164, 179) and in two others, with candidosis and trichosporosis (90, 91). In some cases, epidemiology and in others, the site of the lesions suggested simultaneous infection.

19. Debilitating Factors: Disease and Treatment

In 142 patients of this series — almost three fourth of all cases — other diseases were present.

In 22 cases, no details were mentioned in the reports (100–102, 104, 105–116, 131, 193, 194–197), and in 31 (1–3, 7, 11, 28, 30, 36, 39, 45, 75, 77–79, 81, 91, 117, 134, 144, 147, 152, 153, 158, 159, 164, 165, 168, 182, 185, 186, 192), no debilitating factors were present. Of these, seven had received antibiotics, suggesting that in only 16% of all cases of multiple mycoses other diseases were not present.

In 77 cases, neoplasms were reported. In order of frequency, these included leukemias (more than 50%), Hodgkin's disease, carcinoma, sarcoma, and multiple myeloma. In 32 cases, bacterial infections: pulmonary diseases, tuberculosis, septicemia and others of a more localized nature were reported.

In 18 cases, hematic disorders: anemia, agranulocytosis, leukopenia, myeloesclerosis were seen, and, in 14 renal affections, generally in transplants. Other nonmycotic diseases reported, were 12 cases of intestinal disorders: parasitosis, ulcers, colitis; 8 cases of virosis, generally cytomegaly; 5 cases of diabetes; 4 patients with Protozoan diseases, including toxoplasmosis and Chagas' disease; and 1 case each of SLE, sarcoidosis, Fanconi's syndrome, and rheumatism.

Associations between mycoses and such diseases showed 75% to be invasions by candidosis-aspergillosis, generally in neoplastic diseases, especially leukemia. While the diffuse form of pulmonary aspergillosis occurred most often with debilitating diseases, this was not the case in circumscribed tumorous forms in which local conditions were predisposing factors. Neoplasms, further, were present with all cases of associated geotrichosis and in about one half of the cases of phycomycosis, cryptococcosis, pneumocystosis, and nocardiosis. Aspergillosis and phycomycosis were found associated with hematic disorders. With the 5 cases in which diabetes was the underlying disease, candidosis, phycomycosis, nocardiosis, and histoplasmosis were found. Neither aspergillosis nor cryptococcosis were reported with diabetes.

That treatment may have contributed to the development of multiple fungal infections is suggested by comparison between their increasing incidence (Table 2) and the development of modern therapeutics as listed by Keye and Magee [45]: these authors give the following time table:

1919–1936: Presulfonamide period
1937–1941: Sulfonamide period
1942–1947: Penicillin period
1948–1955: Multiple antibiotics

To which we would add a fifth category: 1956 —: Cytostatics and immuno-suppressive drugs.

Mycoses least frequently found associated with debilitating disorders include histoplasmosis, blastomycosis, paracoccidioidomycosis, the rare and localized fungal infections, and the combination cryptococcosis-candidosis.

When histoplasmosis was observed in debilitating disorders, it was associated with cryptococcosis. The fortuitous association of residual lesions of histoplasmosis and coccidioidomycosis with other mycoses has already been discussed. Blastomycosis was associated generally with histoplasmosis; apparently debilitating diseases played a minor role. In paracoccidioidomycotic infections, the common debilitating factors in populations of tropical countries must be taken into consideration. In the rare and circumscribed fungal infections, as for example cutaneous involvement, the association with other fungal diseases apparently is also fortuitous. No explanation can be given for the fact that the combination of candidosis and cryptococcosis occurred in 50 % of all cases without underlying disease. It may be that a single factor of affinity exists between these two fungus species.

20. Diagnosis and Doubtful Cases

In patients with two mycoses, both were diagnosed during life in 22 %, while only one of the two mycoses was diagnosed in 14 %. Only one case of pneumocystosis was diagnosed in vivo by tracheal aspiration. In 65 % of all cases, neither of the two mycoses had been recognized during life.

In the 15 patients with three fungal infections no information was available on three; in one, the three mycoses were diagnosed during life, in two; two mycoses were diagnosed in vivo. In 9 cases, none of the mycoses was discovered until necropsy. Finally, in a patient with five mycoses, only one fungal infection had been detected before death.

Diagnosis during life has been more frequent in histoplasmosis, blastomycosis, coccidioidomycosis, chromomycosis, and sporotrichosis; less frequent in candidosis, aspergillosis, cryptococcosis, and nocardiosis; and very rare in phycomycosis, pneumocystosis, and geotrichosis. There are several reasons for these differences. One reason is the tendency to focus attention on the management of some obvious disease, without considering the possibility of fungal infections which develop slowly. On the contrary, mycotic infections such as phycomycosis and pneumocystosis develop rapidly or are final complications. Further, in cases where one mycosis is detected, efforts to look for possible concomitant fungal infections may not be made.

11*

Finally, in infections with *Candida* and *Aspergillus*, a single isolation of these species may be regarded often as a saprophytic occurrence, and only if repeated isolations are achieved is the possibility of fungus disease considered.

Since precise information is lacking in quite a few cases, particularly of candidosis, aspergillosis, and geotrichosis, it cannot be said with certainty whether all were true multiple fungus diseases.

In candidosis, Baum [8] rightly insisted that, in addition to cultural proof, histology must reveal tissue lesions. Torack's cases [102] may be accepted, since the fungus was shown to penetrate into the submucosa. Diagnosis of candida infection on histologic grounds alone can be accepted. Exclusive proof by culture, on the other hand (as in cases 7, 48, 73, 85, 86, 90, 91, 124, 157, 158, 162), is not sufficient for diagnosis of mycotic disease.

In the absence of fruit heads, diagnosis of aspergillosis by morphology alone is dubious. In 40 cases, diagnosis was based only on morphology (8, 19, 22, 23, 29, 35, 38, 42–44, 68, 69, 80, 93–95, 97, 99, 118–120, 123, 125–129, 134, 136, 155, 166, 168, 170–176, 178). It was not clear in these cases whether sterigmata with conidia were found or if diagnosis was made only on the basis of demonstration of hyphae. Although dichotomous branching and septate hyphae, which sometimes are not visible in H & E stains, point in the direction of aspergillosis, other fungi, such as *Penicillium*, and others cannot be excluded. In an autopsy study of lungs of healthy as well as of sick persons, *Penicillium sp.* was predominant (Okudaira *et al.* [63]. In cases 88, 89, 124, on the other hand, diagnosis of aspergillosis was based only on culture.

Four of the six cases with geotrichosis were without detailed information, on how diagnosis was achieved, yet it is difficult to differentiate geotrichosis from Candida infection on histologic grounds alone. When septate branching hyphae with typical arthrospores are present, diagnosis may be suspected but needs confirmation by culture (Chang and Buerger [19]).

In addition to the foregoing imprecisely determined cases, eight others in this series must be discussed (2, 7, 76, 84–86, 159, 160), which also seem doubtful from the diagnostic point of view. In cases 2 and 7 (candidosis with cryptococcosis) histologic data are insufficient or lacking. In case 7, a cryptococcosic osteomyelitis was said to have been cured by excision, drainage, and treatment with sulfadiazine, iodides, and an autogenous vaccine. In cases 76 and 86 (penicilliosis with candidosis + pneumocystosis and aspergillosis, respectively), the fungus (*Penicillium*) was isolated in each case and lesions were described only in one tissue. Whether these lesions were attributable to *Penicillium* is an open question.

In cases 84 and 85 (candidosis with cryptococcosis), it is not clear if *Candida* had produced lesions. In addition, in case 85, nests of *Toxoplasma gondii* were described, but no mention is made whether they were Grocott negative (*Histoplasma?*).

In cases 159 and 160 (cryptococcosis with blastomycosis or actinomycosis, respectively), the cryptococcal lesions were not proven as produced by this agent, which had been cultured only from sputum; pulmonary symptoms disappeared without treatment. Nor were actinomycotic lesions described; *Actinomyces* had been cultured only from sputum. The author who describes the case is of the same opinion.

Further, cases 30, 77, 78, 80, and 81 must be considered: In case 30 (histoplasmosis with aspergillosis), diagnosis of histoplasmosis is based only on serology and in the others (histoplasmosis with blastomycosis), diagnosis of both was made only on culture and serology without anatomic evidence. While there is some reason to accept these 5 cases as dual infections, they make clear at least that complete confirmation of multiple fungus infections is laborious and demands the use of as many diagnostic tools as possible. Diagnosis of the histoplasmotic nature of pulmonary cavities should be based on the finding of yeast cells of *H. capsulatum* in the wall of the cavity.

In case 180, taking as evidence only figures 20 and 21 of the first publication (1969), reasonable doubts are raised whether a double generalized fungus infection (paracoccidioidomycosis with histoplasmosis) really existed, as occasionally numerous small, yeastlike cells of *P. brasiliensis* may mimic the cells of *H. capsulatum*, as do also small forms of *B. dermatitidis*. Diagnosis in this case was based exclusively on morphologic grounds and no cultures were made. However, differential diagnosis between these two fungus species can be based exclusively on histologic examination. H & E. stain and the Grocott method do not suffice to establish clearcut morphologic differences which can be photographed; the Gram stain (Weigert's fibrin) is most useful for this purpose. With this method, *P. brasiliensis* cells remain more or less unstained, while *Histoplasma* cells, in contrast, come out heavily dark stained, although their yeast-cell structure is not shown as well as in Grocott-stained preparations.

In mediastinal lymph nodes of this case (180), yeast cells of *P. brasiliensis* and *H. capsulatum* were seen together in the same macrophages or giant cells. In addition, Chagas' disease was present with leishmania nests of *Tr. cruzi* in myocardium and testis (Figs. 1–10).

The present report does not include several cases showing large forms and/or pseudohyphae of *H. capsulatum* in tissues (Binford [11], Schwarz [83], Silverman *et al.* [90] (fourth case), Korns [46], Pinkerton and Iverson [69], Blanchard and Olin [12], Van Breuseghem [107], which may raise the question of infections with an additional fungus species. The atypical large forms of *H. capsulatum*, described by the foregoing authors, were found in necrotic tissues. They do not seem related to the large yeast cells of *H. duboisii* or the "large forms" of *H. capsulatum* in hamster tissue, which have been recognized as Schaumann bodies containing small yeast cells.

Neither have we included cases showing small forms of *B. dermatitidis* in tissues and in which an additional infection with *H. capsulatum* may have been possible (Manwaring [56], Schwarz and Baum [84], Weed [112], Tuttle *et al.* [103], Tompkins and Schleifstein [101]), but was denied by the authors. However, the cases of Manwaring and of Tuttle *et al.* were considered as dual infections (blastomycosis cum histoplasmosis) by the patho-

 K. Salfelder, M. Mendelovici, and J. Schwarz:

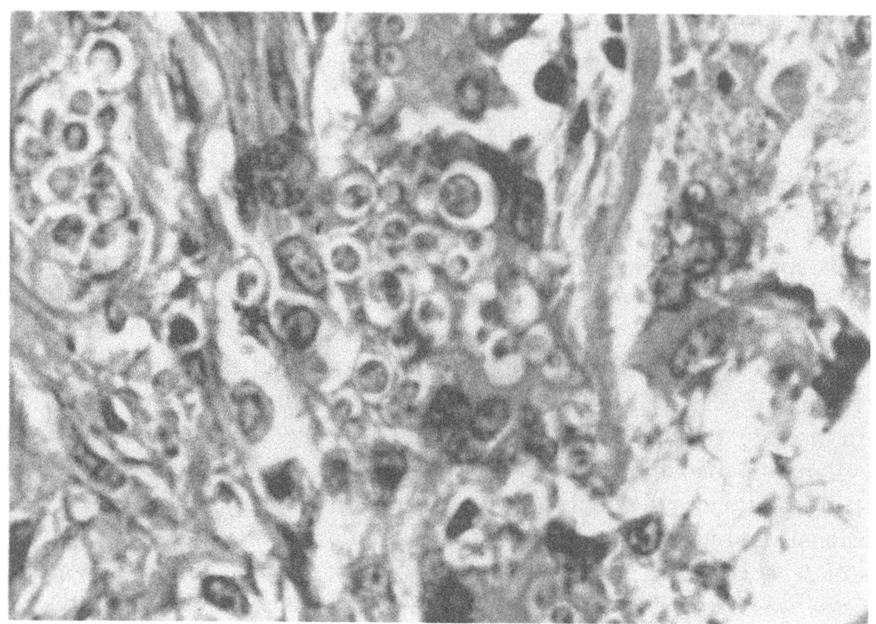

Fig. 1. Case 177, mediastinal lymph node. Only nest of yeast cells of *P. bras.* H & E.; 720 ×

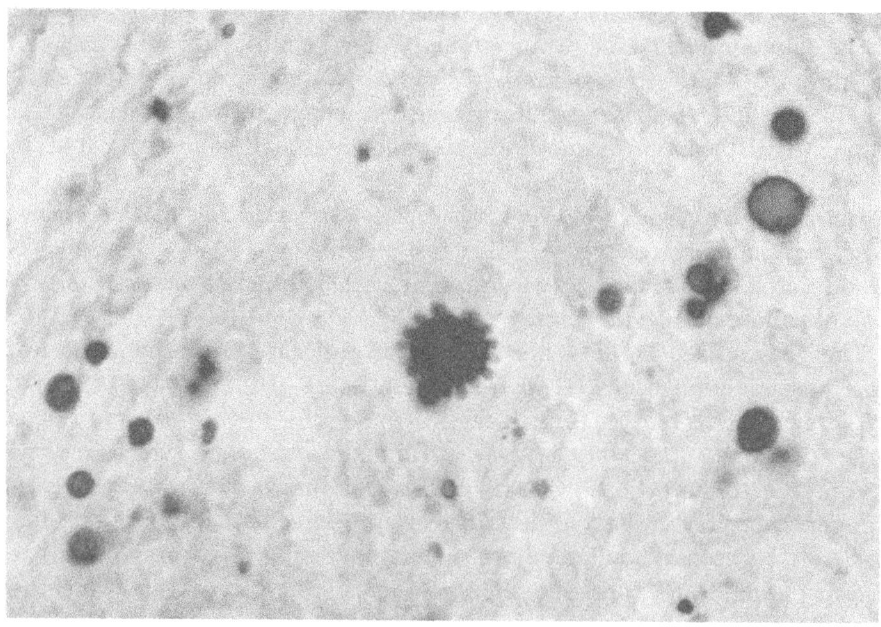

Fig. 2. Case 177, mediastinal lymph node. Steering-wheel form (multiple budding) of a yeast cell of *P. bras.* Grocott method; 1150 ×

logists of the Armed Forces Institute of Pathology in Washington DC (Layton *et al.* [49], Brandsberg *et al.* [14]). The figures of Manwaring's paper are suggestive of a dual infection.

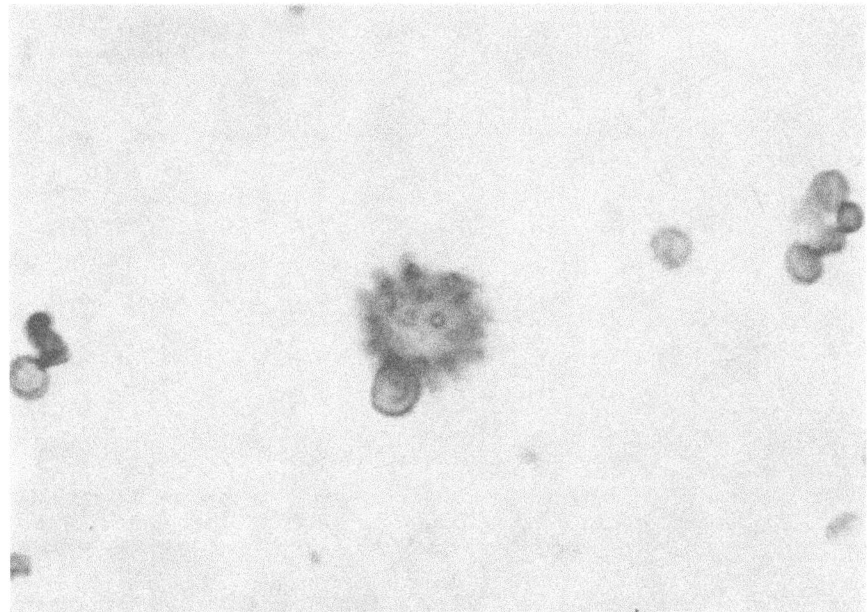

Fig. 3. Case 177, mediastinal lymph node. Same yeast cell as in Fig. 3 focused at another level to show buds distributed over entire surface

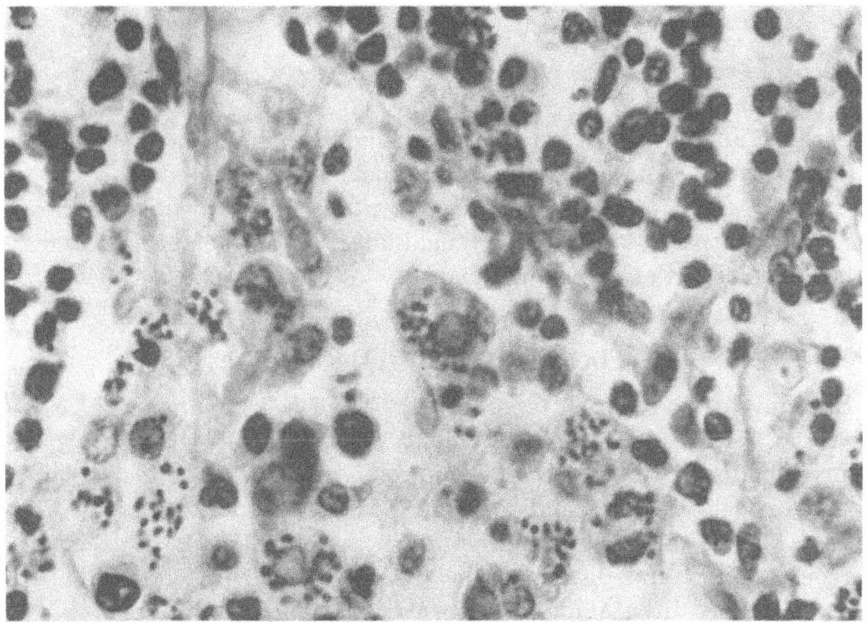

Fig. 4. Case 177, mediastinal lymph node. Yeast cells of *H. capsulatum*, mostly intra-cellular. H & E.; 720 ×

Two other cases (chromomycosis + blastomycosis and/or histoplasmosis, reported by ALMEIDA and LACAZ (1939) and chromomycosis + actinomycosis, reported by NEVES DA SILVA (1949), cited by BOPP and LIMA [13] are not

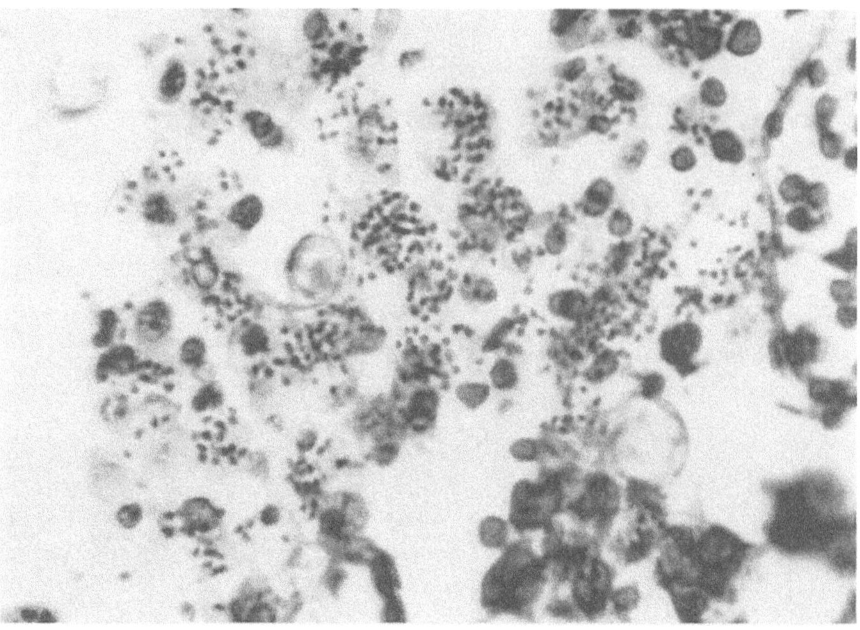

Fig. 5. Case 177, mediastinal lymph node. Yeast cells of *P. bras.* and *H. capsulatum* in same field. *H. capsulatum* darkly stained, *P. bras.* faintly. Fibrin staining (Gram-Weigert); 720 ×

included, as reprints were not available and the description by Bopp and Lima is not conclusive.

Case 2 of Fors and Sääf [31] was not included. In a pulmonary "mycetoma" with quite broad septate dichotomous branching hyphae and spores in tissue sections, *Candida albicans* and *Candida tropicalis* were grown in cultures. The case was not considered as double fungal infection by the authors. It may be an aspergilloma with *Candida* infection.

21. Therapy for Multiple Mycoses

Dual mycoses have been reported to respond well to amphotericin B (34, 36, 40, 192), with some variability of effectiveness in a few cases. In patients with meningitis as well as coccidioidomycosis, administration of amphotericin B must be long-term; in candidosis, no evidence of cure had been reported.

Total dosage and long-term therapy with amphotericin B is important to avoid relapses and dissemination (191). An inadequately treated histoplasmosis shows little improvement over untreated histoplasmosis (CDC, CMS [21]). Some mycoses, for instance histoplasmosis, may need higher total doses of amphotericin B than others. In cases where treatment has been interrupted due to severe reactions, dissemination of one or both mycoses has been observed (46).

Because of the possible toxic effects (renal damage) of amphotericin B therapy, patients receiving this drug require especially careful management.

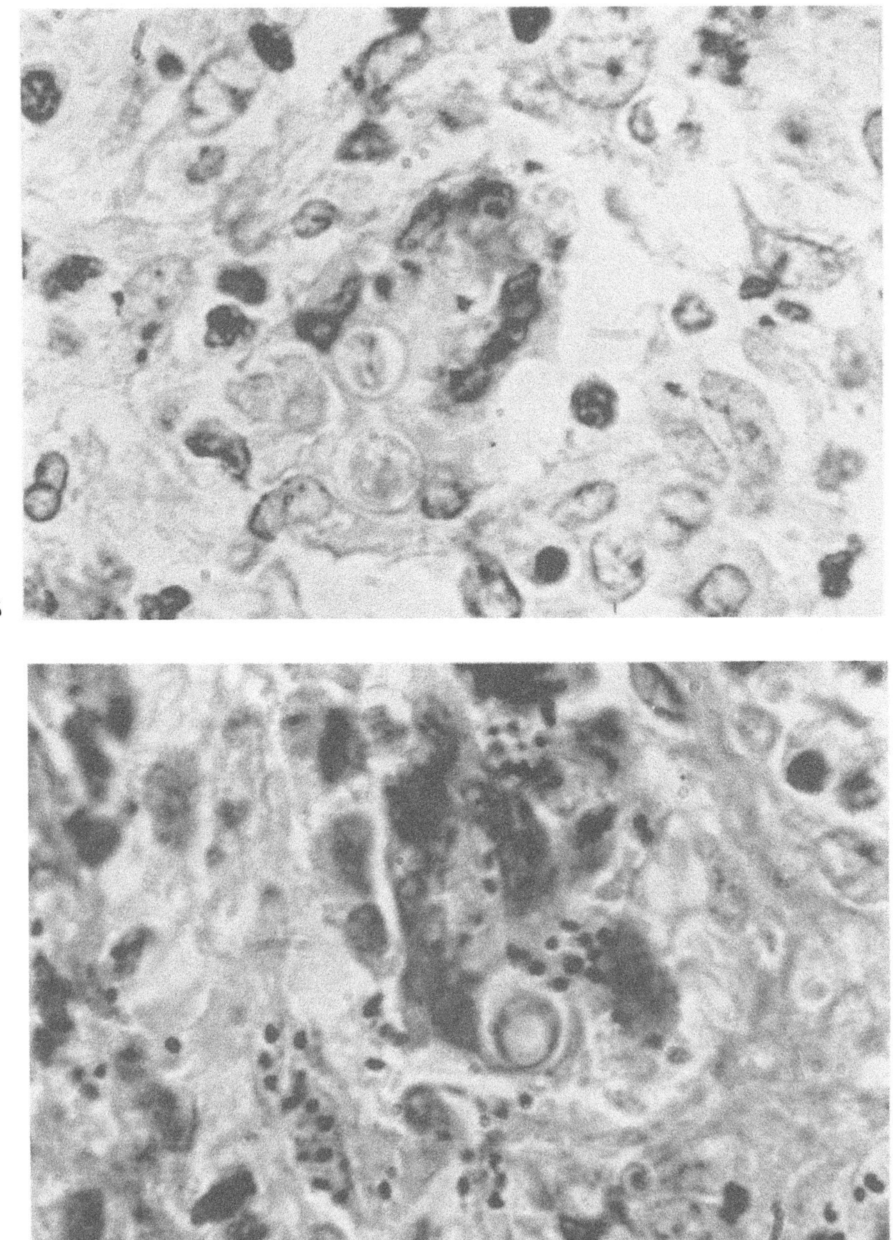

Fig. 6 and 7. Case 177, mediastinal lymph node. Yeast cells of *P. bras.* and *H. capsulatum* together in giant cells. Fibrin staining (Gram-Weigert); 1150 ×

Several fungus infections have responded well to specific therapy other than amphotericin B. Aspergillomas are reportedly sensitive to inhalation of nystatin, and nocardiosis responds well to antibiotics. In pneumocystosis, amphotericin B was of no use (154, 160), but recently a case responded to a pen-

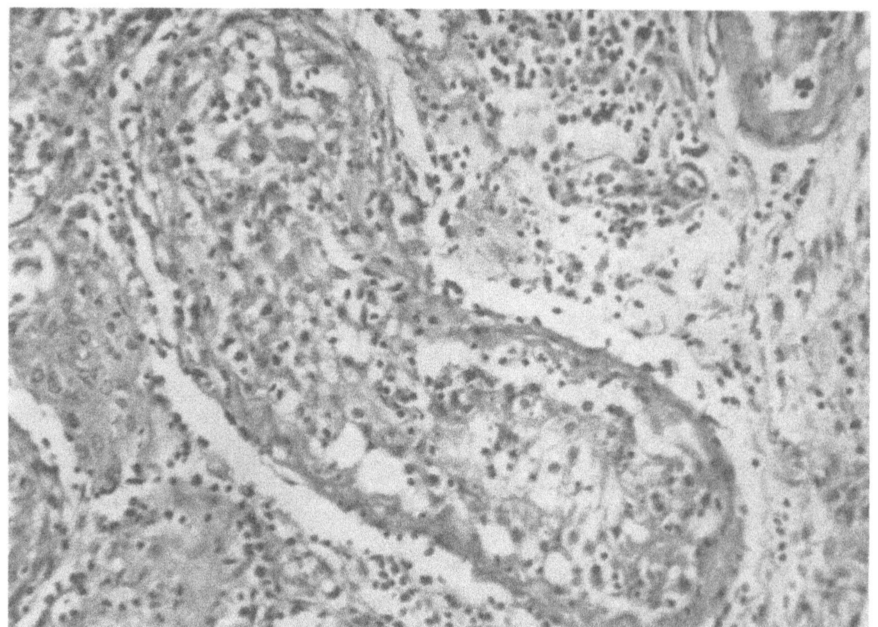

Fig. 8. Case 177, testis. Marked orchitis. Organisms faintly visible inside of tubules. H & E.; 190 ×

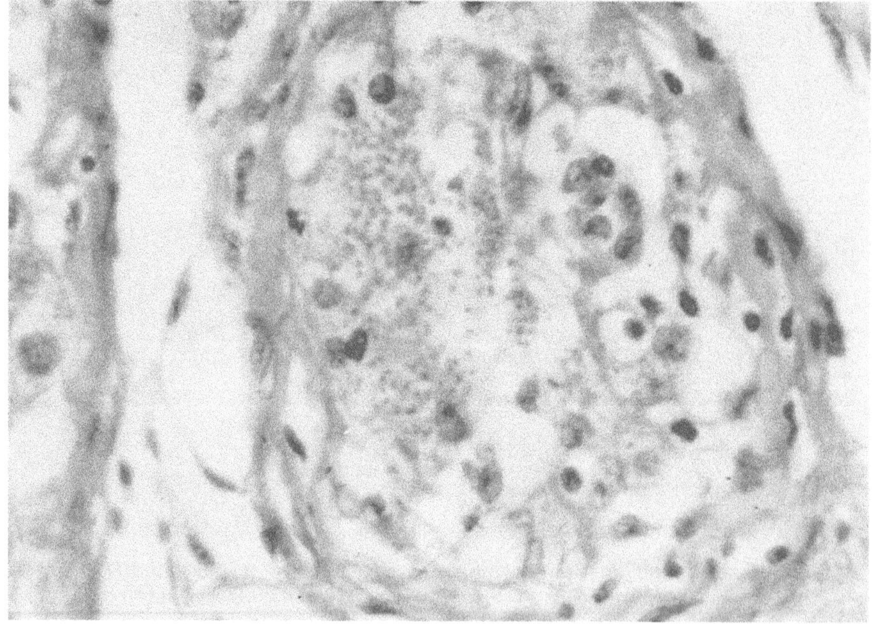

Fig. 9. Case 177, testis. Chagas' orchitis. Leishmania forms clearly visible inside of tubules (Grocott-negative). H & E.; 600 ×

tamidine derivate (FORTUNY *et al.* [32]). Surgery has been effective in tumorous and localized lesions.

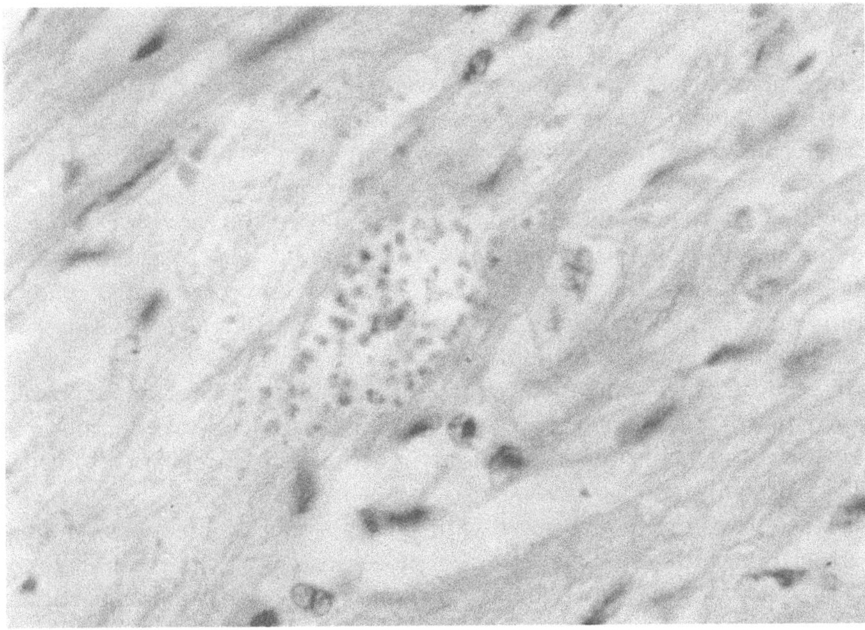

Fig. 10. Case 177; myocardium. Nest of leishmanias in muscle fiber. H & E.; 750 ×

D. Summary and Conclusions

Multiple fungus infections in 201 cases are reviewed, with data from 184 reported in the literature and 13 unpublished cases. Two additional cases involved infections with several species of *Aspergillus* and two others were of blastomycosis, in which a secondary infection with *H. capsulatum* may be assumed, though not acknowledged by the authors. The period covered is from 1947 to 1970, during which time the incidence of reports of such infections has been greatly increased. All except 16 cases involved dual infections; of these, 15 involved triple and 1 a quintuple fungal infection.

Spontaneous multiple fungus infection in animals was not commented on since we know only of one such case: dual infection by histoplasmosis and blastomycosis in a dog (MENGES *et al.* [58]).

Cases were reported from only 9 countries, a few papers containing the bulk of the casuistics. Reports of numerous cases are generally from cancer hospitals.

Data on relation to race or occupation were inadequate for conclusions to be drawn. The male sex predominated, several of the mycoses being reported only in males.

Fifty percent of the patients were over age 45, and actinomycosis, nocardiosis, blastomycosis, coccidioidomycoses, paracoccidioidomycosis, chromomycosis, sporotrichosis, and mycetoma were reported only in adults.

In more than three-fourths of all cases, autopsies were either reported or assumed to have been performed. All cases involving phycomycosis, pneumocystosis, nocardiosis, and geotrichosis were autopsied.

The most frequent associations were candidosis-aspergillosis and aspergillosis-phycomycosis. No-affinity or antagonism could be found between cryptococcosis and aspergillosis + phycomycosis. Blastomycosis occurred only with histoplasmosis. In rare associations, a fortuitous coincidence can be supposed; also in combinations with residual histoplasmotic and coccidioidal lesions in endemic areas. In the cases with more than two mycoses similar conditions were found. Mycoses not found associated with other fungal infections were: rhinosporidiosis, African histoplasmosis, Lobo's Disease.

In almost three-fourths of all cases, debilitating diseases apparently favored fungal infection. Previous diseases were generally neoplasms (more than 50% were leukemias), bacterial infections, hematologic disorders, or renal transplants.

Diabetes was rarely associated with multiple fungus infections, and never in association with aspergillosis or cryptococcosis.

The validity of diagnosis in many instances can be questioned, particularly when it is based only on morphology in tissues. We feel strongly that conclusive diagnosis should be based on culture, and only exceptionally, in experienced hands, is morphology alone adequate for diagnosis. On the other hand, it is safe to assume that many cases of multiple mycoses are overlooked in treating more prominent and obvious conditions. In cancer and hematology services, variable percentages were indicated (Gerszten et al. [36]: 1,5; Pedraza [65]: 2,5; Miyake and Okudaira [60]: 3,5; Hutter and Collins [43]: 7 and Pedraza [65]: 7,5 %).

It seems strange that in reports treating a high number of mycoses not a single dual or multiple fungal infection was mentioned (Ahn Changwoo et al. [2], Benaim Pinto [9], Berdnikoff [10], Butler et al. [17], Withorsh and Utz [118], Lacaz [47]).

We believe that the combination of blastomycosis and histoplasmosis is more frequent than has yet been recognized. With the constantly increasing interstate travel in the United States and intercountry travel abroad, it would be nothing less than strange if increasing incidence of multiple fungal infections did not occur.

Finally, the physician who finds one mycosis should lower his threshold of suspicion of the possibility that another fungal infection may well be present, and should be governed accordingly in his examination of the patient.

References

1. Abbott, J. D., Fernando, H. V. J., Gurling, K., Meade, B. W.: Pulmonary aspergillosis following post-influenzal bronchopneumonia treated with antibiotics. Brit. med. J. 1952I, 523–525.
2. Ahn Changwoo, Kilman, J. W., Vasko, J. S., Andrews, N. C.: The therapy of cavitary pulmonary histoplasmosis. J. thorac. cardiovasc. Dis. 57, 42–51 (1969)

3. ALKIEWICZ, J. A., JEWOZA, L., JANIAKOWA, E.: Hefebefunde im Duodenum bei Kindern und Säuglingen. Mykosen **13**, 311–314 (1970).
4. ALLISON, F., LANCASTER, M. G., WHITEHEAD, A. E., WOODBRIDGE, H. B.: Simultaneous infection in man by *Histoplasma capsulatum* and *Blastomyces dermatitidis*. Amer. J. Med. **32**, 476–489 (1962).
5. ANGULO ORTEGA, A., RODRIGUEZ, C., GARCIA GALINDO, G.: Criptococcosis in Venezuela. Mycopath. Mycol. appl. **30**, 367–388 (1961).
6. BAKER, R. D.: Leukopenia and therapy in leukemia as factors predisposing to fatal mycoses: Mucormycosis, aspergillosis and cryptococcosis. Amer. J. clin. Path. **37**, 358–373 (1962).
7. BARNETT, R. N., HULL, J. G., VORTEL, V., SCHWARZ, J.: Pneumocystis carinii in lymph nodes and spleen. Arch. Path. **88**, 175–180 (1969).
8. BAUM, G. D.: The significance of *Candida albicans* in human sputum. New Engl. J. Med. **263**, 70–73 (1960).
9. BENAIM PINTO, H.: La Paracoccidioidomycosis brasiliensis como enfermedad sistemática. Mycop. Mycol. appl. **15**, 90–114 (1961).
10. BERDNIKOFF, G.: Fourteen personal cases of Pneumocystis carinii pneumonia. Canad. med. Ass. J. **80**, 1–5 (1959).
11. BINFORD, C. H.: Histoplasmosis: tissue reactions and morphologic variations of the fungus. Amer. J. clin. Path. **25**, 25–36 (1955).
12. BLANCHARD, A. J., OLIN, J. S.: Histoplasmosis with sarcoid-like lesions occurring in multiple myeloma. Canad. med. Ass. J. **85**, 307–311 (1961).
13. BOPP, C., LIMA, G. M.: Tríplice Infecção Micótica: Cromoblastomicose associada á Blastomicose de Lutz e á Esporotricose. Med. Cir. **18**, 35–45 (1957).
14. BRANDSBERG, J. W., TOSH, F. E., FURCOLOW, M. L.: Concurrent infection with *Histoplasma capsulatum* and *Blastomyces dermatitidis*. New Engl. J. Med. **270**, 874–877 (1964).
15. BRASS, K.: Las micosis profundus. Jornadas Dr. Ramón Arcay Tortolero. Valencia. Diciembre 1966, p. 31–88.
16. BRASS, K.: Mucor-Meningo-Encephalitis basalis und Lungenhistoplasmom eine tuberkulöse Infektion vortäuschend. Mykosen **13**, 165–170 (1970).
17. BUTLER, W. T., ALLING, D. W., SPICKARD, A., UTZ, J. P.: Diagnostic and prognostic value of clinical and laboratory findings in cryptococcal meningitis. A follow-up study of 40 patients. New Engl. J. Med. **270**, 59–67 (1964).
18. CAMPOS DE MAGELHÃES, M. J.: Blastomicosis por *Blastomyces dermatitidis* am Africa. Apresentação do primeiro caso em Mocambique. I Congresso Nacional de Anatomia Patológica, Universidad de Lourenco Marques, 863–877, 1968.
19. CHANG, W. W. L., BUERGER, L.: Disseminated geotrichosis. Arch. intern. Med. **113**, 356–360 (1964).
20. CLARK, B. M.: Epidemiology of phycomycosis. In: WOLSTENHOLME, G. E. W., and PARKER, R., eds., Systemic mycoses. London: J. & A. Churchill 1968.
21. Communicable Disease Center Cooperative Mycoses Study. Comparison of treated and untreated severe Histoplasmosis. J. Amer. med. Ass. **183**, 823–829 (1963).
22. CROSS, R. M., BINFORD, C. H.: Infections by fungi that are commonly primary pathogens. Is Nocardia asteroides an opportunist? Lab. Invest. **11**, 1103–1109 (1962).
23. DOEHNERT, G., DOEHNERT, H. R., LISCANO, T. R. DE, GONZALEZ, R., SALFELDER, K.: La Neumocistosis en Venezuela. Trib. med. **264**, 9–23 (1968).
24. DOEHNERT, G., DOEHNERT, H. R., SALFELDER, K.: Dreifachinfektion mit *Paracoccidioidoides brasiliensis*, *Trypanosoma cruzi* und *Histoplasma capsulatum*. Z. Tropenmed. Parasit. **21**, 202–209 (1970).
25. DRUTZ, D. J., SPICKARD, A., ROGERS, D. E., KOENIG, M. G.: Treatment of disseminated mycotic infections. A new approach to amphotericine B therapy. Amer. J. Med. **45**, 405–418 (1968).
26. EMMONS, C. W., MURRAY, I. G., LURIE, H. I., KING, M. H., TULLOCH, J. A., CONNOR, P. H.: North American blastomycosis: two autochtonous cases from Africa. Sabour. **3**, 306–311 (1964).
27. EMMONS, C. W., BINFORD, L. H., UTZ, J. P.: Medical mycology, 2d. ed. Philadelphia: Lea & Febiger 1970.

28. Esterly, J. A., Warner, N. E.: *Pneumocystis carinii* pneumonia. Twelve cases in patients with neoplastic lymphoreticular disease. Arch. Path. **80**, 433–441 (1965).
29. Falcone, M. W., Garagusi, V. F.: Sporotrichosis and nocardiosis in a patient with Boeck's disease. S. Med. J. **3**, 315–318 (1969).
30. Finegold, S. M., Will, D., Murray, J. F.: Aspergillosis. A review and report of twelve cases. Amer. J. Med. **27**, 463–482 (1959).
31. Fors, B., Sääf, J.: Localized pulmonary mycosis. A problem of diagnosis. (Report of 4 cases treated by resection.) Acta chir. scand. **119**, 212–229 (1960).
32. Fortuny, F. E., Tempero, K. F., Amsden, T. W.: *Pneumocystis carinii* pneumonia diagnosed from sputum and successfully treated with pentamidine isothionate. Cancer (Philad.) **26**, 911–913 (1970).
33. Frenkel, J. K.: Pathogenesis of infections of the adrenal gland leading to Addison's disease in man; the role of corticoids in adrenal and generalized infections. Ann. N. Y. Acad. Sci. **84**, 391–440 (1960).
34. Furcolow, M. L.: Opportunism in histoplasmosis. Lab. Invest. **11**, 1134–1139 (1962).
35. Gemeinhardt, H.: Zur Frage der Pathogenität des Sproßpilzes *Trichosporon capitatum* im Respirationstrakt des Menschen. Ein Beitrag zur Diagnostik der Lungenmykosen. Z. Tuberk. **124**, 190–197 (1965).
36. Gerszten, E., Allison, M. J., Dalton, H. P.: A ten year study of mycotic infections in a Virginia General Hospital. Amer. J. clin. Path. **52**, 445–450 (1969).
37. Gilbert, C. F., Fordham, C. C., Bemson, W. R.: Death resulting from *Pneumocystis* pneumonia in an adult. Arch. inter. Med. **112**, 158–163 (1963).
38. Gowing, N. F. C., Hamlin, I. M. E.: Tissue reactions to Aspergillus in cases of Hodgkin's disease and leukemia. J. clin. Path. **13**, 396–413 (1960).
39. Gruhn, J. G., Sanson, J.: Mycotic infections in leukemic patients at autopsy. Cancer (Philad.) **16**, 61–73 (1963).
40. Hendry, W. S., Patrick, R. L.: Observations on thirteen cases of *Pneumocystis carinii* pneumonia. Amer. J. clin. Path. **38**, 401–405 (1962).
41. Hill, R. B., Rowlands, D. T., Rifkind, D.: Infections pulmonary diseases in patients receiving immunosuppressive therapy for organ transplantation. New Engl. J. Med. **271**, 1021–1027 (1964).
42. Hutter, R. V. P.: Phycomycetous infection (Mycormycosis) in cancer patients; a complication of therapy. Cancer (Philad.) **12**, 330–350 (1959).
43. Hutter, R. V. P., Collins, H. S.: The occurrence of opportunistic fungus infections in a cancer hospital. Lab. Invest. **11**, 1035–1045 (1962).
44. Jarnum, S., Rasmussen, E. F., Ohlsen, A. S., Sorensen, A. W. S.: Generalized *Pneumocystis carinii* infection with idiopathic hypoproteinemia. Ann. intern. Med. **68**, 138–145 (1968).
45. Keye, J. D., Magee, W. E.: Fungal diseases in a general hospital: study of 88 patients. Amer. J. clin. Path. **26**, 1235–1253 (1956).
46. Korns, M. E.: Coincidence of mycotic (*Histoplasma capsulatum*) vegetative endocarditis of the mitral valve and the Lutembacher syndrome. Circulation **32**, 589–592 (1965).
47. Lacaz, C. S.: South American blastomycosis. An. Fac. Med. Univ. São Paulo **29**, 1–20 (1955–1956).
48. La Touche, C. J., Sutherland, T. W., Telling, M.: Rhinocerebral mucormycosis. Lancet, **1963 II**, 811–813.
49. Layton, J. M., McKee, A. P., Stamler, F. W.: Dual infection with *Blastomyces dermatitidis* and *Histoplasma capsulatum*. Report of a fatal case in man. Amer. J. clin. Path. **23**, 904–913 (1953).
50. Ledebur, C. D., von: Contribution à l'étude des mycoses cérébrales humaines. (11 cas anatomo-cliniques.) Thèse n° 2981, Facultéde Médecine, Genève, Suisse, 1968.
51. Leggat, P. O., Kretser, D. M. de: Aspergillus pneumonia in association with an aspergilloma. Brit. J. Dis. Chest. **62**, 147–150 (1968).
52. Leopold, S. S.: Pulmonary moniliasis and cryptococcal osteomyelitis in the same patient. Med. Clin. N. Amer. **37**, 1737–1747 (1953).
53. Levy, S. E., Cohen, D. B.: Systemic moniliasis and aspergillosis complicating corticotropin therapy. Arch. intern. Med. **95**, 118–122 (1955).
54. Magaldi, C., Amato Nato, V., Marchioni Monteiro, D. C.: Criptococcose. Rev. Hosp. Clin. F. Med. São Paulo **19**, 19–32 (1964).

55. MAHNKE, P. F., ZCHOSCH, H., SIECHERT, H.: Pilzbefunde im Tracheobronchialbaum des Menschen. Häufigkeit, Arten und Pathogenetische Bedeutung. Path. Microb. **24**, 327–340 (1961).
56. MANWARING, J. H.: Unusual forms of *Blastomyces dermatitidis* in human tissues. Arch. Path. **48**, 421–425 (1949).
57. McCARTHY, D. S., LONGBOTTOM, J. L., RIDDELL, R. W., BATTEN, J. C.: Pulmonary mycetoma due to *Allescheria boydii*. Amer. Rev. resp. Dis. **100**, 213–216 (1969).
58. MENGES, R. W., McCLELLAN, J. T., AUSHERMAN, R. J.: Canine histoplasmosis and blastomycosis in Lexington, Kentucky. J. Amer. vet. med. Ass. **124**, 202–207 (1954).
59. MIDER, G. B., SMITH, F. D., BRAY, W. E.: Systemic infection with *Cryptococcus neoformans* (Torula histolytica) and *Histoplasma capsulatum* in the same patient. Arch. Path. **43**, 102–110 (1947).
60. MIYAKE, M., OKUDAIRA, M.: A statistical survey of deep fungus infections in Japan. Acta path. jap. **17**, 401–415 (1967).
61. MORRIS, J. H., MacAULAY, M., POSER, C. M.: Systemic cryptococcis and histoplasmosis in the same patient. Neurology (Minneap.) **14**, 147–153 (1964).
62. MOSBERG, W. H., ARNOLD, J. G.: Torulosis of the central nervous system. Review of literature and report of five cases. Ann. intern. Med. **23**, 1153–1183 (1950).
63. OKUDAIRA, M., KURATA, H., SAKABE, F., SOPEDA, M.: (A study on the fungal flora in the lung of human necropsy cases.) Jap. J. Med. Mycol. **6**, 231–251 (1965).
64. PARKER, J. D., SAROSI, G. A., DOTO, I. L., TOSH, F. E.: Pulmonary aspergillosis in sanatoriums in the South Central United States. Amer. Rev. resp. Dis. **101**, 551–557 (1970).
65. PEDRAZA, M. A.: Mycotic infections at autopsy. A comparative study in two university hospitals. Amer. J. clin. Path. **51**, 470–476 (1969).
66. PEÑA, C. E.: Deep mycotic infections in Colombia: a clinico-pathologic study of 162 cases. Amer. J. clin. Path. **47**, 505–520 (1967).
67. PERRY, L. V., JENKINS, D. E., WHITCOMB, F. C.: Simultaneously occurring pulmonary coccidioidomycosis and histoplasmosis. Amer. Rev. resp. Dis. **92**, 952–957 (1965).
68. PILLAY, V. K. G., WILSON, D. M., TODD, S., KARK, R. M.: Fungus infection in steroid treated systemic Lupus erythematosus. J. Amer. med. Ass. **205**, 261–265 (1968).
69. PINKERTON, H., IVERSON, L.: Histoplasmosis. Three fatal cases with disseminated sarcoidlike lesions. Arch. intern. Med. **90**, 456–467 (1952).
70. POLLAK, L., ANGULO ORTEGA, A.: Las micosis broncopulmonares en Venezuela. Tórax. **16**, 135–145 (1967).
71. PREISLER, H. D., HASENCLEVER, H. F., LEVITAN, A. A., HENDERSON, E. S.: Serologic diagnosis of disseminated Candidiasis in patients with acute leukemia. Ann. intern. Med. **70**, 19–30 (1969).
72. PROCKNOW, J. J., LOEWEN, D. F.: Pulmonary aspergillosis with cavitation secondary to histoplasmosis. Amer. Rev. resp. Dis. **82**, 101–111 (1960).
73. RANKIN, N. E.: Disseminated aspergillosis and moniliasis associated with agranulocytosis and antibiotic therapy. Brit. med. J. **1953I**, 918–919.
74. RIFKIND, D., FARIS, T. D., HILL, R. B.: *Pneumocystis carinii* pneumonia. Studies on the diagnosis and treatment. Ann. intern. Med. **65**, 943–956 (1966).
75. ROCHA POSADA, H., MARTIN, F., MÉNDEZ LEMAITRE, A.: Histoplasmosis systemática. Macopath Mycol. appl. **36**, 55–74 (1968).
76. RODGER, R. C., TERRY, L. L., BINFORD, C. H.: Histoplasmosis, cryptococcosis and tuberculosis complicating Hodgkin's disease. Amer. J. clin. Path. **21**, 153–157 (1951).
77. ROSEN, P., ADELSON, H. T., BURLEIGH, E.: Bronchiectasis complicated by the presence of *Monosporium apiospermum* and *Aspergillus fumigatus*. Amer. J. clin. Path. **52**, 182–187 (1969).
78. SAENZ JIMENEZ, L., MORERA, P.: Sobre un caso de Blastomicosis sur-americana asociada a cromonicosis. Acta med. Costa Rica **6**, 55–71 (1963).
79. SALFELDER, K., LISCANO, T. R. DE, GONZÁLEZ, R., CARLESSO, J.: Pauciparasitic pneumocystosis. Mykosen **10**, 589–592 (1967).
80. SALFELDER, K., DOEHNERT, G., DOEHNERT, H. R.: Paracoccidioidomycosis. Virchows Arch. Abt. A. **348**, 51–76 (1969).

81. Salfelder, K., Brass, K., Doehnert, G., Doehnert, H. R., Sauerteig, E.: Fatal disseminated histoplasmosis. Virchows Arch. Abt. A. **350**, 303–335 (1970).
82. Saltzman, H. A., Chick, E. W., Conant, N. F.: Nocardiosis as a complication of other diseases. Lab. Invest. **11**, 1110–1117 (1962).
83. Schwarz, J.: Giant forms of *H. capsulatum* in tissue explants. Amer. J. clin. Path. **23**, 898–903 (1953).
84. Schwarz, J., Baum, G. L.: Blastomycosis. Amer. J. clin. Path. **21**, 999–1029 (1951).
85. Schwarz, J., Baum, G. L.: Fungus diseases of the lungs. Semin. in Roentg. **5**, 3–84 (1970).
86. Schwarz, J., Baum, G. L., Straub, M.: Cavitary histoplasmosis complicated by fungus ball. Amer. J. Med. **31**, 692–700 (1961).
87. Sethi, K., Salfelder, K., Schwarz, J.: Pulmonary fungus flora in experimental pneumocystosis of cortisone-treated rats. Mycopath. Mycol. appl. **24**, 121–129 (1964).
88. Sichert, H., Mahnke, P. F.: Hefe-Oekologie des Trachealbaumes. Zbl. Bakt. **170**, 562–568 (1960).
89. Sidransky, H., Pearl, M. A.: Pulmonary fungus infections associated with steroid and antibiotic therapy. Dis. Chest. **39**, 630–642 (1961).
90. Silverman, F. N., Schwarz, J., Lahey, M. E., Carson, R. P.: Histoplasmosis. Amer. J. Med. **19**, 410–459 (1955).
91. Soper, R. T., Silber, D. L., Holcomb, G. W.: Gastrointestinal histoplasmosis in children. J. pediat. Surg. **5**, 32–39 (1970).
92. Spicer, C., Hiatt, W. O., Kessel, J. F.: *Candida albicans* and *Cryptococcus neoformans* occurring as infective agents in an eight year old boy. J. Pediat. **33**, 761–769 (1948).
93. Straatsma, B. R., Zimmerman, L. E., Gass, J. D.: Phycomycosis. A clinico-pathological study of 51 cases. Lab. Invest. **11**, 963–985 (1962).
94. Straub, M., Schwarz, J.: Primary arrested lesions of coccidioidomycosis and histoplasmosis. A study of autopsy material in Tucson, Arizona. Amer. J. clin. Path. **26**, 998–1009 (1956).
95. Straub, M., Fishkin, B. G., Schwarz, J.: Residual pulmonary lesions of fungal origin in Southern California. Mycopath. Mycol. appl. **20**, 55–59 (1963).
96. Symmers, W. St. C.: Further cases of exotic mycoses seen in Britain. Histoplasmosis, chromomycosis, rhinosporodiosis and phycomycosis. Trans. roy. Soc. trop. Med. Hyg. **55**, 201–208 (1961).
97. Symmers, W. St. C.: Generalised cytomegalic inclusion-body disease associated with pneumocystosis pneumonia in adults. J. clin. Path. **13**, 1–21 (1960).
98. Symmers, W. St. C.: Infections as complications of drug therapy. Exc. Med. Int. Congr., ser. **85**, 108–151 (1965).
99. Symmers, W. St. C.: Septicaemic candidosis. Symposium on Candida infections. 196–213, 1966.
100. Symmers, W. St. C.: Deep fungal infections currently seen in the histo-pathologic service of a medical school laboratory in Britain. Amer. J. clin. Path. **46**, 514–537 (1966).
101. Tompkins, V., Schleifstein, J.: Small forms of *Blastomyces dermatitidis* in human tissues. Arch. Path. **55**, 432–435 (1953).
102. Torack, R. M.: Fungus infections associated with antibiotics and steroid treatment. Amer. J. Med. **22**, 872–882 (1957).
103. Tuttle, J. G., Lichtwardt, H. E., Altschuler, C. H.: Systemic North American blastomycosis. Report of a case with small forms of blastomycetes. Amer. J. clin. Path. **23**, 890–897 (1953).
104. Tynes, B., Mason, K. M., Jennings, A. E., Benneth, J. E.: Variant forms of pulmonary cryptococcis. Ann. intern. Med. **69**, 1117–1125 (1968).
105. Utz, J. P., Andriole, V. T., Emmons, C. W.: Chemotherapeutic activity of X5079C in systemic mycoses of amn. Amer. Rev. resp. Dis. **84**, 514–528 (1961).
106. Utz, J. P.: The spectrum of opportunistic fungus infections. Lab. Invest. **11**, 1018–1025 (1962).
107. van Breuseghem, R.: *Histoplasma Duboisii* and large forms of *Histoplasma capsulatum*. Mycologia 48, 264–269 (1956).
108. van Breuseghem, R.: With the collaboration of J. Coremans-Pelsencer D. Swinne-Desgain and A. Janssens-Van Dyck.: Post-mortem investigation of 100 cancerous patients. Mykosen **13**, 337–350 (1970).

109. VIVIAN, D. N., WEED, L. A., McDONALD, J. R., CLAGETT, O. T., HODGSON, C. H.: Histoplasmosis: clinical and pathological study of 20 cases. Surg. Gynec. Obstet. **99**, 53–62 (1954).
110. WAHNER, H. W., HEPPER, N. G. G., ANDERSON, H. A., WEED, L. A.: Pulmonary aspergillosis. Ann. intern. Med. **58**, 472–485 (1963).
111. WALZ, D. V., HASENCLEVER, H. F., McKEE, A. P.: A dual human infection with *Candida albicans* and *Cryptococcus neoformans*. Amer. J. clin. Path. **26**, 794–798 (1956).
112. WEED, L. A.: Large and small forms of blastomyces and histoplasma. Amer. J. clin. Path. **23**, 921–923 (1953).
113. WELSCH, R. A., BUCHNESS, J. M.: Aspergillus endocarditis, myocarditis and lung abscesses. Report of a case. Amer. J. clin. Path. **25**, 782–786 (1955).
114. WHITTAKER, R. H.: New concepts of kingdoms of organisms. Science **163**, 150–160 (1969).
115. WILL, D. W., MURRAY, J. F., FINEGOLD, S. M., SUTTER, V. L., FISHKIN, B. F.: Dissemination of coccidioidomycosis in patients with neoplastic diseases. Amer. Rev. resp. Dis. **84**, 114 (1961).
116. WINN, W. R., FINEGOLD, S. M., HUTTINGTON, R. W.: Coccidioidomycosis with fungemia. 2d Coccid. Symp. Phoenix, Ar. 93–109, 1967.
117. WINSLOW, D. J., HATHAWAY, B. M.: Pulmonary pneumocystosis and cryptococcosis. Report of a case of mixed infection in a United States adult. Amer. J. clin. Path. **31**, 337–342 (1959).
118. WITHORSH, PH., UTZ, J. P.: North American blastomycosis: a study of 40 patients. Medicine (Baltimore) **47**, 169–200 (1968).
119. YOUNG, R. C., BENNETT, J. E., VOGEL, C. L., CARBONE, P. P., DE VITA, V. T.: Aspergillosis. The spectrum of the disease in 98 patients. Medicine (Baltimore) **49**, 147–173 (1970).
120. ZIMMERMAN, L. E., RAPPAPORT, H.: Occurrence of cryptococcosis in patients with malignant disease of the reticulo-endothelial system. Amer. J. clin. Path. **24**, 1050–1072 (1954).

Author Index

Page numbers in *italics* refer to bibliography. Numbers shown in square brackets
are the numbers of the references in the bibliography

12*

Index to Volumes 37—56

Ergebnisse der allgemeinen Pathologie und der pathologischen Anatomie

Current Topics in Pathology

Current Topics in
Pathology

Ergebnisse der Pathologie

Reprint from

Vol. 57

Morphology and Pathogenesis of
Glomerulopathy in Cadaver Kidney
Allografts Treated with Antilymphocyte
Globulin
(Clinical, Light, Electron and Immunofluo-
rescent Optic Examinations)

H. U. Zollinger, J. Moppert, G. Thiel,
H.-P. Rohr

With 42 Figures

Springer-Verlag Berlin · Heidelberg · New York 1973

Current Topics in Pathology

Ergebnisse der Pathologie

Reprint from

Vol. 57

Some Aspects of Sarcoidosis

Henry A. Azar, Edward A. Moscovic,
Solange G. AbuNassar,
J. Steven McDougal

With 14 Figures

Springer-Verlag Berlin · Heidelberg · New York 1973

Current Topics in
Pathology

Ergebnisse der Pathologie

Reprint from

Vol. 57

The Interepithelial Lymphocytes of the
Intestinum. Morphological Observations
and Immunological Aspects
of Intestinal Enteropathy

H. F. Otto

With 14 Figures

Springer-Verlag Berlin · Heidelberg · New York 1973

Current Topics in Pathology

Ergebnisse der Pathologie

Reprint from **Vol. 57**

Multiple Deep Fungus Infections:
Personal Observations and a Critical
Review of the World Literature

K. Salfelder, M. Medelovici, J. Schwarz

With 10 Figures

Springer-Verlag Berlin · Heidelberg · New York 1973

Hypertension '72

**Edited by
Jacques Genest and Erich Koiw**

Symposium, organized by the Clinical Research Institute of Montreal, under the auspices of the University of Montreal Medical School

304 figures. XVI, 617 pages. 1972. Soft cover DM 88,—; US $27.90

The essential features of this book are the important and new contributions concerning the basic disturbances of aldosterone regulation in benign essential hypertension, the discovery of isoenzymes of renin in brain and arterial tissue, independent of the renal renin system, the discovery of a new ß-converting enzyme in submaxillary glands, a discussion-in-depth of the mechanisms controlling renin release and of the disturbances of mineralocorticoid hormones other than aldosterone in benign essential hypertension.

**Springer-Verlag
Berlin Heidelberg New York**

London München Paris Sydney Tokyo Wien

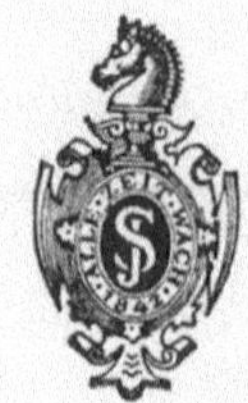

Universitätsdruckerei H. Stürtz AG, Würzburg

GPSR Compliance
The European Union's (EU) General Product Safety Regulation (GPSR) is a set
of rules that requires consumer products to be safe and our obligations to
ensure this.

If you have any concerns about our products, you can contact us on

ProductSafety@springernature.com

In case Publisher is established outside the EU, the EU authorized
representative is:

Springer Nature Customer Service Center GmbH
Europaplatz 3
69115 Heidelberg, Germany